www.GlutenFreeDietBook.com

presents

Gluten Free-Easy

Second Edition

Easy Recipes

that are Gluten-Free

(not Taste-Free)

ISBN: 978-1-84799-783-8

Table of Contents

INTRODUCTION

So you've been diagnosed as suffering from celiac (coeliac) disease or as gluten-intolerant - or there's no firm diagnosis yet, but you've been advised to try going gluten free for a few weeks to see if this fixes your health problem.

Or possibly you are going gluten free off your own bat, because you aren't getting anywhere with professionals and your research indicates it might be gluten that is causing your health problems.

Now that you've been taken up this challenge, you're beginning to realize that it's quite a big deal: so many foods we eat every day without thinking contain gluten, and not just the ones that are obvious, either.

You started trying to work out which foods you can't eat, but really you're beginning to think it would be easier to make a list of the things you CAN eat! It looks as if you need to cut out almost all pre-packed and processed foods for a start. Things are looking desperate - what are you going to eat?

WHERE DOES GLUTEN COME FROM?

Gluten is found in the protein portion of wheat, rye and barley. Another very similar compound is found in oats, so you may need to exclude these as well (though not all who are gluten-intolerant have a problem with oats).Other grains which may cause a problem are spelt (a primitive form of wheat) and triticale (a hybrid wheat).

The gluten is the part of the grain which gives it its 'stretchiness', what gives bread its texture. Non-gluten 'breads' are available, but they are often much more like cake, more crumbly and without the 'mouth feel' of normal bread.

Even though gluten is only in the protein part, it is not safe to eat any portion of the grains which contain it (including oats if you are affected by oat-'gluten'), because there will be a certain amount of gluten still present.

WHO NEEDS TO BE GLUTEN FREE?

If you've been diagnosed with gluten-sensitive enteropathy, coeliac disease, non-tropical sprue, coeliac sprue, primary malabsorption, ideopathic steatorrhoea or dermatitis herpetiformis, you are strongly gluten intolerant and need to cut it out of your diet altogether.

It's possible you are gluten-intolerant if you have these problems:

Other conditions which are possibly linked to gluten intolerance include: autism, depression, diabetes, infertility, irritable bowel syndrome (IBS), multiple sclerosis, regional enteritis, rheumatoid arthritis, schizophrenia and Sjögren's syndrome.

Common symptoms of gluten-intolerance are: flatulence ('wind') after eating gluten; abdominal distension; stools ('poos') which are pale, bulky, greasy and smelly; diarrhoea; headache; nausea and vomiting; poor appetite and drowsiness after eating; muscle cramps and spasms; bone or joint pains; anaemia, with weight loss; any of the symptoms listed flaring up under stress; obesity; oedema (puffy swollen legs); or constipation.

Your best option if you suffer from any of the conditions listed (or one or more of the symptoms in the second paragraph) is to try living gluten free for a few weeks, and see if the situation improves. If it does, try eating a small amount of gluten, and watch for a reaction. Be prepared for it to be greater than you expect!

IF YOUR CHILD IS GLUTEN INTOLERANT

Kids want to be like everybody else. I guess we all have that to some degree, but to a child, it's very important for their self-esteem that they don't stand out from the crowd. For an adult, having to cut out gluten is a nuisance, but to a child, it can be far more than that.

Once they start school, your children will want to bring their friends home for tea and what you serve up may make all the difference between them making firm friends who will come round to play regularly, or not. If they make friends, of course, they will also be receiving invitations to tea at their friends' houses.

You need to talk to the school, and also teach your child what they can eat, and what they can't. It's no good imposing a blanket ban on 'sweets from strangers,' as sooner or later, these get disobeyed.Without the knowledge only you can give them, they will not have the ability to distinguish what is safe from what is not. It is very likely that some well-meaning but ignorant substitute teacher, friend or friend's parent will give them something that they should not be eating, so they do need to be aware.

When your child gets an invitation to a friend's house, you need to assess the parents. Have a chat to them about your child's diet. If you have any doubt as to their ability to comply with it, you would be best to offer to feed both children first, and send them round to play afterwards.

All the recipes in this book are suitable for children, of course, but there are some that are particularly likely to be appreciated, and I have marked these with the label **Recipes Kids Love** and moved them to the end of each section for ease of reference. It's perfectly possible that your kids will like the other recipes just as much, or even better - and most of the recipes selected for children will go down just as well with adults.

ABBREVIATIONS USED IN THIS BOOK

in or "	inch/es
oz	ounce/s
fl oz	fluid ounce/s
lb	pound/s
tsp	teaspoon/s (about 5ml)
tblsp	tablespoon/s (about 15ml)
g	gram/s
kg	kilogram/s
ml	millilitre/s
GF	gluten free

CHECK ALL ingredient labels EVERY TIME YOU BUY

BASICS

Pastry 1
180g (6 oz) potato flour
60g (2 oz) rice flour
120g (4 oz) butter or margarine, softened
90g (3 oz) caster sugar
1 egg

Put all ingredients into a bowl and work together until a dough is formed.

Dust with rice flour. Wrap in foil - flatten into a block about 2.5cm (1") thick and chill in fridge overnight. Use like standard pastry - can be frozen for up to 3 months.

Pastry 2
90g (3 oz) rice flour
60g (2 oz) potato flour
30g (1 oz) soy flour
pinch of salt
90g (3 oz) butter or margarine
1 egg, beaten

Rub the fat into the flour, pour in the egg and mix. well Use as required, or roll into a flan case and bake blind for 10 mins at 200° C (400° F, gas mark 6), then fill as required.

Pie crust 1
350g (12 oz) yellow maize meal (polenta)
½ tsp salt
3 tblsp oil
about 150ml (¼ UK pint, $\frac{5}{8}$ US cup) hot stock

Mix the dry ingredients with enough stock to make a stiff better.

Pat into a 22.5 cm deep pie dish.
Add your preferred filling and continue with recipe.

CHECK ALL ingredient labels EVERY TIME YOU BUY

Pie crust 2

2 cups cooked brown rice
2 tblsp butter
1 beaten egg
180g (6 oz) grated Parmesan
Juice of 1 lemon
30g (1 oz) sesame seeds

Preheat oven to 180°C, (350°F, gas mark 4).

Grind sesame seeds in a blender to make a coarse meal - take it slow, and don't overdo it or you will end up with sesame butter (tahini).

Melt butter, mix with egg, parmesan, lemon juice and sesame seeds. Mix into rice.

Pat into a pie tin and bake for 10 minutes.

Continue with your recipe.

Panbread/pan pizza base

1 cup gluten free flour
1 egg
a pinch of salt (optional)
$\frac{1}{3}$ cup of water (more or less as required)

Break egg into flour and salt, and knead together into rather sticky "breadcrumbs".

Add water, sufficient to make a sticky dough.

Break into 3 pieces.

Flour the worktop and flatten the dough into the size required. You will probably need to reflour a couple of times before you have finished this step.

Cook one at a time in an oiled pan over a low to medium heat, turning once.

Serve immediately or leave to cool and serve same day, the fresher the better.

CHECK ALL ingredient labels EVERY TIME YOU BUY

Bread 1

Makes 3 small (1lb) loaves

175g (6 oz, 1 US cup) brown rice
500ml (¾ UK pint, 2 US cups) water
1 tblsp honey
250g (8 oz) soy flour
250g (8 oz) maize flour
250g (8 oz) rice flour
30g (1 oz) fresh yeast *or* 15g (½ oz) dried yeast
½ tblsp sunflower oil
450ml (¾ UK pint, 1 US pint) water which has been used
 for boiling potatoes

Cook the rice with the 2 cups of water and honey until the water is absorbed.

Mix together the cooked rice, all the flours, the oil and salt. Dissolve the yeast in the potato water and mix into flour and rice mixture to make a dough.

Divide between 3 small (1lb) loaf tins and leave for 30 minutes in a warm place.

Preheat oven to 180° C (350° F, gas mark 4) while the loaves are resting.

Bake for approximately 45 minutes.

Remove from tins and leave to cool.

CHECK ALL ingredient labels EVERY TIME YOU BUY

Bread 2

Makes 1 small loaf

180g (6 oz) maize flour
90g (3 oz) rice flour
1½ tsp gluten free baking powder
1 tsp salt
60g (2 oz) butter or margarine
1 egg
250ml (8 fl oz, 1 US cup) milk

Preheat oven to 200° C (400° F, gas mark 6).

Grease a 15cm (6") loaf tin.

Mix all ingredients together, and pour into the tin, bake for 25 to 30 mins.

Home made almond paste ('Marzipan')

Makes enough to cover a 20 cm (8") cake

350g (12 oz) ground almonds
175g (6 oz) caster sugar
3 egg whites
2-3 drops almond essence
3 tblsp jam, without fruit

Mix almonds and sugar. Beat egg whites with almond essence and add to mixture. Blend to form a paste. Knead well.

Marzipanning a cake

Divide mixture in half. Shape and roll out half to a circle about 1 cm (¼") larger than the top of the cake. Brush top of cake with warmed jam. Place circle of almond paste onto the cake and smooth down.

Measure the height of the sides of the cake ("A") and the circumference ("B"). Roll out remaining paste into an oblong as wide as "A", and as long as "B".

Brush the sides of the cake with jam and press on strips of marzipan, joining neatly. Either leave plain to ice, or pinch with fingers to decorate.

CHECK ALL ingredient labels EVERY TIME YOU BUY

Royal icing

Makes enough to cover a 20 cm (8") cake

4 egg whites
1 kg (2 lb) icing sugar, sieved
20ml (4 tsp) lemon juice
10ml (2 tsp) glycerine

Whisk egg whites until frothy. Stir in icing sugar gradually, beating well until smooth, stiff and shiny. Stir in lemon juice and glycerine.

Icing a cake

Spoon a dollop of icing on top of the cake and spread evenly over the surface, using a backwards and forwards motion with the knife. With a palette knife or ruler scrape off the surplus to smooth over top. Spread icing round sides using palette knife to smooth. Trim edges.

Using a piping bag with a star shaped nozzle no 6, pipe a scallop shell edging around the top of the cake. Use the same icing mix to stick decorations (e.g. bride and groom, Father Christmas, etc.) to the top of the cake. For a Christmas cake, tie a large red ribbon round the cake, and stick with a couple of dabs of icing.

CHECK ALL ingredient labels EVERY TIME YOU BUY

SOUPS AND STARTERS

Red bean soup

6 Servings

450g (15 oz) can red kidney beans
1-2 cloves garlic, crushed
4 tblsp olive oil
Salt and pepper

Pour half the beans into a saucepan, purée the remainder in a food processor. Taste and adjust seasoning. Add to whole beans in pan.

Sauté chopped garlic in the olive oil until golden. Add to soup, bring to the boil and serve.

Artichoke soup

8 Servings

4 tblsp olive oil
1 large onion, finely chopped
750ml (1½ UK pints, $3\frac{7}{8}$ US cups) chicken stock*
350ml (12 fl oz, 1½ US cups) dry white wine
2 garlic cloves, crushed
600g (1½ lb) Jerusalem artichokes, finely chopped
½ tsp salt
¼ tsp black pepper
2 level tblsp fresh chives, chopped
125ml (4 fl oz, ½ US cup) double (heavy) cream or
     crème fraîche
parsley for garnish

Heat oil in large pan and fry onion until golden.

Add stock, wine and garlic and bring to the boil.

Add artichokes, reduce heat, simmer for 20 minutes.

Remove from the heat. Blend until smooth and creamy. Season to taste.

Reheat and serve with 1 tblsp cream or crème fraîche on top of each bowl, garnished with parsley.

* For a vegetarian version, substitute vegetable stock for chicken stock.

CHECK ALL ingredient labels EVERY TIME YOU BUY

Scallop chowder
4-6 Servings

30g (1 oz) butter
1 medium onion, sliced thinly
2 sticks celery, chopped
2 medium carrots, diced
1 large potato, diced
125g (4 oz) lean bacon, chopped
275ml (½ UK pint, 1¼ US cups) vegetable stock
350g (12 oz) white fish fillets, skinned and cubed
125g (4 oz) scallops, sliced
275ml (½ UK pint, 1¼ US cups) milk
1 tblsp cornflour (cornstarch) or arrowroot
Salt and pepper
Chopped parsley to garnish

Sauté onion, celery, carrot, potato and bacon until onion is transparent.

Add stock and simmer until potatoes are tender.

Add fish and scallops and simmer for 4 minutes only.

Blend milk and cornflour or arrowroot and add to pan in a thin stream, stirring continuously. Stir until thickened.

Serve garnished with parsley.

Brussels sprout soup
4 Servings

500g (1 lb) Brussels sprouts
570ml (1 UK pint, 2½ US cups) stock
1 small onion, sliced
2 tblsp single cream
salt and black pepper
nutmeg to taste (optional)

Prepare sprouts, add to a pan with the chicken stock and cook gently until tender (20-25 minutes). Cool and liquidize.

Return to pan, heat gently (but not to boiling point). Add cream and season to taste. Serve.

CHECK ALL ingredient labels EVERY TIME YOU BUY

Crab soup
4-6 Servings

30g (1 oz) butter (or 1 tblsp oil)
1 large onion, chopped
400g (13½ oz) can tomatoes, chopped
600ml (21 fl oz) fish or chicken stock
225g (7½ oz) sweetcorn (corn kernels)
or 125g (4 oz) mushrooms, chopped
350g (12 oz) crab meat
1 tblsp cornflour (cornstarch) or arrowroot
Salt and pepper
Chopped parsley to garnish

Sauté onion gently in the butter or oil until transparent, add tomatoes, cover and simmer for 5 minutes.

Add stock, sweetcorn or mushrooms and crab meat. Cover and simmer for a further 3 minutes.

Blend milk and cornflour or arrowroot and add to pan in a thin stream, stirring continuously. Stir until thickened.

Serve garnished with parsley.

Bouillabaise
6-8 Servings

2 tblsp olive oil
1 large onion, sliced
1 clove garlic, crushed
2x400g (13½ oz) cans tomatoes, chopped
900ml (1½ UK pints, 3¾ US cups) fish or chicken stock
2 tblsp chopped parsley
Salt and pepper
1 bouquet garni*
500g (1 lb) monkfish, diced
500g (1 lb) redfish fillet, skinned and diced
350g (12 oz) coley fillet, skinned and diced
350g (12 oz) catfish fillet, skinned and diced
600g (1¼ lb) plaice fillet, skinned and cut into strips

Sauté onion and garlic until soft.

CHECK ALL ingredient labels EVERY TIME YOU BUY

Stir in tomatoes, stock, parsley, salt and pepper. Add bouquet garni. Bring to the boil and simmer for 10 minutes.

Add all the fish except the plaice and simmer for 5 minutes.

Add plaice and simmer for a further 5 minutes.

Remove bouquet garni and serve, garnished with a little more chopped parsley.

* A bouquet garni is traditionally a bunch of herbs tied together which is cooked with the dish but removed before serving, so that the flavor remains but no leaves are left in the dish. The standard ingredients are parsley, thyme and a bay leaf. However, other ingredients may be used either as additions or on their own. You can buy ready made bouquets garnis in little muslin bags, or just use a pinch of each herb, and a bay leaf.

Borschch (Russian beetroot soup)
8-10 Servings

1.5kg (3 lb) cooked beetroot, diced
2 stalks celery chopped
1 large onion, finely chopped
2 litres (3½ UK pints, 9 US cups) beef stock
500g (1 lb) cabbage, shredded
1 tsp salt
1½ tsp black pepper
2 bay leaves
2 tblsp wine vinegar
250ml (8 fl oz, 1 US cup) sour cream
2 tblsp parsley, chopped

Combine beetroot, celery and onion in a large pan. Add sugar and stock to cover. Bring to the boil, ensuring sugar dissolves. Cover and simmer for 20 minutes, stirring occasionally.

Add cabbage, simmer for 20 minutes.

Pour in remaining stock, salt, pepper, bay leaves and vinegar. Lower heat and cook for about 20 minutes. Remove bay leaves. To serve stir 1 tblsp sour cream into each bowl and sprinkle with parsley.

CHECK ALL ingredient labels EVERY TIME YOU BUY

Celery and Stilton soup
4 Servings

1 head of celery with leaves
2 medium onions
60g (1 oz) butter
900ml (1½ UK pints, 3¾ US cups) chicken stock
150ml (¼ UK pint, $\frac{5}{8}$ US cup) milk
125g (4 oz) white Stilton cheese
3 tblsp double (heavy) cream
Salt and pepper

Reserve the best looking celery leaves for garnish and chop the rest, along with the stalks. Chop onion. Sauté together in the butter very gently for about 10 minutes.

Add chicken stock, bring to the boil and adjust seasoning. Simmer for 30 minutes.

Allow to cool for a few minutes, then transfer to a blender or food processor in batches, blending until smooth. Sieve out the celery fibres and return to pan, adding the milk.

Mash cheese into a soft paste with the cream.

Heat soup to just below boiling point and stir 2 tblsp of the hot soup into the creamed cheese. Pour the cheese mixture back into the pan, stirring continuously.

Check and adjust seasoning and serve garnished with the reserved celery leaves.

Buttermilk soup
6 Servings

250g (8 oz) cooked shrimps or prawns, shelled
half a cucumber
1 tblsp fresh dill
1 tblsp made mustard
1 tsp salt
1 tsp sugar
1 litre (1¾ UK pints, 4½ US cups) buttermilk

Chop the dill, cucumber and shrimps or prawns. Put in a

CHECK ALL ingredient labels EVERY TIME YOU BUY

blender with the mustard, salt and sugar. Blend until smooth.

Stir in the milk, chill and serve.

Lentil soup
6 Servings

175g (6 oz) lentils
1 clove garlic, crushed
175g (6 oz) cooking bacon, diced
1 onion, chopped
1 large carrot, diced
1 litre (1¾ UK pints, 4½ US cups) water

Put all the ingredients into a large cooking pot. Bring to the boil, cover and lower heat to a simmer.

Cook for about 20 minutes, stirring occasionally until the lentils have become completely soft and easy to mash.

Allow to cool for a few minutes, then transfer in batches to a food processor or blender and blend until smooth.

Return to pan, reheat, check seasoning and serve.

Chilled prawn soup
6 servings

570ml (1 UK pint, 2½ US cups) plain gluten free yogurt
570ml (1 UK pint, 2½ US cups) tomato juice
Half a cucumber
1 tsp lemon juice
Salt and pepper
180g (6 oz) cooked peeled prawns
Chopped chives to garnish

Blend yogurt, tomato juice, cucumber, lemon juice and half the prawns together in a food processor or blender until fairly smooth. Check and adjust seasoning.

Transfer to the serving bowls, dividing the remaining prawns equally. Chill.

Garnish with chopped chives before serving.

CHECK ALL ingredient labels EVERY TIME YOU BUY

Avocado mousse

4 Servings

2 ripe avocado pears
2 tblsp lemon juice
1 tblsp olive oil
150ml (¼ UK pint, $\frac{5}{8}$ US cup) double (heavy) cream
small pinch of sugar (optional)
salt and pepper

Cut avocados in half, remove stones and scoop out flesh. Blend with lemon juice.

Stir in olive oil and lemon juice gradually, beating to mix well.

Pile back into the avocado shells, garnish with parsley and serve chilled.

RECIPES KIDS LOVE

Chicken and bamboo shoot soup
8 Servings

8 large or 16 small mushrooms
1 tblsp oil
1 clove garlic, crushed
2 tsp fresh ginger, peeled and finely chopped
2 raw chicken breasts, thinly sliced
1.5 litres (2½ UK pints, 6½ US cups) chicken stock
125g (4 oz) bamboo shoot, thinly sliced
salt and pepper
125g (4 oz) uncooked Kenya (needle) beans, whole
2 spring (green) onions, sliced

If you can get dried Chinese mushrooms, these are the best. Alternatively, use straw mushrooms (available in tins from Chinese supermarkets), oyster mushrooms or ordinary mushrooms (in order of preference).

If using dried mushrooms, put them into cold water to cover and soak for 1 hour. Squeeze dry.

Slice mushrooms thinly, removing hard parts, if present.

Heat oil in pan, fry garlic and ginger together for 1 minute until browning. Add mushrooms and cook for a further 1-2 minutes.

Stir in chicken. Add stock and bamboo shoot. Season, bring to the boil and simmer for 2-3 minutes.

Top and tail the beans and add to the soup. Simmer for another 3-5 minutes.

Stir in onions and serve hot.

CHECK ALL ingredient labels EVERY TIME YOU BUY

Pakora
6-8 Servings

2 large potatoes, peeled and cut into small pieces
1 onion, chopped coarsely
1 cup gram flour (besan/chickpea flour/garbanzo flour)
½ cup water
1 teaspoon red chilli powder (more or less, to taste)
4 cloves of crushed garlic
7.5 cm (3 inches) of crushed ginger
a pinch of salt
2 tblsp chopped fresh coriander
Oil for frying

A fast and easy starter or side dish for an Indian meal, or a popular snack for kids, but you will probably need to omit or reduce the chilli in this case.

Mix gram flour, salt and water to a batter, mix in the other ingredients.

Heat about 2.5cm of oil in a deep frying pan and add spoonfuls of the mixture. Cook until golden, turning so that they are cooked on all sides.

Drain on kitchen towel and serve hot or cold. Good with dip made from yogurt, mint sauce and more chilli.

You can vary this by using a greater variety of vegetables, such as mushrooms, courgettes (zucchini), sweet peppers, cauliflower florets, bhindi (lady's fingers), aubergine (eggplant) etc.

Summer soup
4 Servings

30g (1 oz) butter
1 lettuce
250g (8 oz) peas (fresh or frozen)
250ml (8 fl oz, 1 US cup) stock
125ml (4 fl oz, ½ US cup) single cream
2 tblsp chives, finely chopped
salt and pepper

CHECK ALL ingredient labels EVERY TIME YOU BUY

Wash lettuce, break into individual leaves. Melt butter in saucepan. Add lettuce and cook for 1 minute, turning frequently.

Add peas and stock. Bring to the boil, stirring, and simmer for 15 minutes.

Blend. Chill.

Serve with a swirl of cream and a sprinkling of chopped chives on the top of each bowl.

Beetroot soup
4 Servings

500ml (¾ UK pint, 2 US cups) stock
1 small onion, finely chopped
150g (6 oz) cooked beetroot, coarsely chopped
3 level tsp cornflour (cornstarch) or arrowroot
125ml (4 fl oz, ½ US cup) milk
1-2 tblsp gluten free horseradish sauce
salt and black pepper
1 carton gluten free natural yogurt

Cook the onion in the stock until soft, about 5-7 minutes. Add beetroot and bring to the boil. Turn off the heat.

Blend the cornflour or arrowroot with milk to a smooth cream. Pour in a steady stream into the pan, stirring continuously until the mixture thickens.

Add horseradish sauce, salt and pepper. Simmer for 2 minutes. Serve with 2 tblsp yogurt swirled into each serving.

CHECK ALL ingredient labels EVERY TIME YOU BUY

Creamy celery soup

4 Servings

1 large head of fresh celery, coarsely chopped
1 large potato, cooked and diced
salt and black pepper
¼ tsp dried tarragon
60g (2 oz) quartered button mushrooms
pinch nutmeg
125ml (4 fl oz, ½ US cup) single cream
725ml (1¼ UK pints, 3¼ US cups) water

Simmer the celery in the salted water for 30 minutes.

Liquidize celery and liquid together and return to pan.
Add tarragon, mushrooms, potato and nutmeg and
simmer for 2-3 minutes. Check seasoning, stir in cream
and serve.

Tomato sorbet

4 Servings

60g (2 oz) caster sugar
500ml (¾ UK pint, 2 US cups) water
2 egg whites
400ml (13½ oz) can tomatoes
½ tblsp tomato purée
¼ tsp Tabasco sauce
2 tsp Worcestershire sauce
salt and black pepper

Combine sugar and water in a saucepan. Heat gently to
dissolve sugar. Cool. Liquidize tomatoes and add to
sugar water with the other ingredients, mix well.

Pour into a shallow plastic box with a fitting lid. Put into
freezer and leave for about 2-4 hours until just freezing.

Stiffly whip egg whites.

Turn sorbet into a bowl and mash with a fork until
smooth. Fold in egg whites. Put back into the container
and store in the freezer until required. Use within 3
months.

CHECK ALL ingredient labels EVERY TIME YOU BUY

MAIN COURSES: MEAT BASED

Devilled kidneys
4 Servings

500g (1 lb) lambs' kidneys, skinned, cored and sliced
250g (½ lb) mushrooms, sliced
100g (3 oz) melted butter
1½ tsp Worcestershire sauce (preferably Lea & Perrin's)
2 tblsp lemon juice
1 tblsp French mustard
parsley to garnish

Sauté kidneys and mushrooms in the butter until tender, about 5 minutes.

Mix the other ingredients together and add to the pan. Simmer for 3 minutes. Check seasoning.

Serve on a bed of rice, garnished with parsley.

Piquant pork
6 Servings

6 large pork chops
180g (6 oz) cooking apple, cut in rings
1 large sliced onion
2 sliced tomatoes
60g (2 oz) butter
½ tsp dried or 1 tblsp fresh tarragon

Preheat oven to 170°C (350°F, gas mark 4).

Lay chops in the bottom of a baking dish greased with 1 tblsp of the butter, cover with apple slices, chopped onion and tomatoes. Dot with remaining butter and sprinkle with tarragon.

Cover and cook for 45 minutes until meat is tender. Drain off cooking juices and serve.

CHECK ALL ingredient labels EVERY TIME YOU BUY

Beef in oyster sauce
8 Servings

500g (1 lb) rump or fillet steak
2 tblsp oil
4 slices fresh root ginger
2 cloves garlic, crushed
2 spring (green) onions, sliced
5 tblsp gluten free oyster sauce
250g (½ lb) French (green/stick) beans, topped and
    tailed

Marinade:
1 level tsp salt
1 level tsp caster sugar
1 tblsp rice wine or dry sherry (optional)
12 tsp oil
2 level tsp cornflour (cornstarch) or arrowroot
½ tsp pepper
2 egg whites

Combine all marinade ingredients in a bowl, mixing well.
Shred steak into thin strips and add, turning to ensure all
the meat is covered. Cover and refrigerate for at least 1
hour, or overnight.

Remove steak from marinade and pat dry on kitchen
towel. Heat oil in pan and fry meat, stirring, for 1-2
minutes. Remove and keep hot.

Sauté ginger and garlic for 2-3 minutes, add onions and
beans and cook for a further 1-2 minutes.

Add meat and oyster sauce and mix well. Serve hot.

Liver Stroganoff
4 Servings

60g (2 oz) butter
2 tblsp oil
1 large onion, thinly sliced
60g (2 oz) mushrooms, sliced
2 large tomatoes, peeled, de-seeded and chopped

CHECK ALL ingredient labels EVERY TIME YOU BUY

500g (1 lb) calves' or lambs' liver
275ml (½ UK pint, 1¼ US cups) sour cream
salt and pepper

Heat butter and oil in a frying pan and fry the onions gently until soft and golden.

Add the mushrooms and tomatoes and cook for 2 minutes.

Slice the liver into thin slivers, about 7-8cm x 1cm (3" x ½") thick. Add to pan and cook, turning mixture over, for a further 5 minutes.

Stir in sour cream and heat through. Check seasoning and serve with potatoes or rice and green salad.

Cabbage patch special
6-8 Servings

a white cabbage, about 2 kg (4 lb) in weight
1 kg (2 lb) mince
2 large onions, finely chopped
200ml (7 oz) can tomatoes
400ml (13½ oz) can red kidney beans
125g (4 oz) mushrooms, chopped
2 tsp chilli powder
salt and pepper

Remove outer leaves of cabbage and discard. Cut the stalk side to make a firm base. Cut a lid about 7-8cm (3") from the top of the cabbage and set aside. Scoop out most of the centre of the cabbage, leaving a shell about 2cm (¾") thick all round.

Cook the mince, onions, chopped tomatoes, mushrooms, salt and pepper into a saucepan. Wash off the beans, drain and add to the pan. Cook for 10-15 minutes.

In another pan, cook the cabbage base and lid in plenty of salted water for about 15 minutes. Drain well.

Put the cabbage on a serving dish and fill with the mince mixture, piling any excess around the base. Put the lid on and serve.

CHECK ALL ingredient labels EVERY TIME YOU BUY

Poulet Provençale

4 Servings

4 chicken portions
125g (4 oz) mushrooms
30g (1 oz) butter
1 large onion, finely chopped
1 clove garlic, crushed
400ml (13½ oz) can tomatoes, drained
½ tsp Herbes de Provence or mixed herbs
salt and pepper
275ml (10 fl oz) can condensed kidney soup
or 400ml (13½ fl oz) can kidney soup

Make sure you check that the soup is gluten free.

Preheat oven to 180°C (350°F, gas mark 4).

Skin chicken.

Fry mushrooms in butter for 2 minutes, add onions and garlic, fry until golden. Transfer to a casserole dish.

Fry chicken until browned.

Add chicken, tomatoes and seasoning to the casserole dish. Pour kidney soup over. If using condensed soup, add half a can of water (or the same quantity of juice from the tomatoes).

Cover and bake for 1½ hours. Serve.

Flemish hearts casserole

4 Servings

3 lambs' hearts
60g (2 oz) streaky bacon, chopped
1 medium onion, chopped
1 tsp Demerara (Turbinado) sugar
275ml (½ UK pint, 1¼ US cups) brown ale
juice of half a lemon
1 bay leaf
pinch of celery salt
salt and pepper

CHECK ALL ingredient labels EVERY TIME YOU BUY

Preheat oven to 170°C (325°F, gas mark 3).

Wash hearts, trim off gristle and excess fat. Cut roughly into cubes.

Fry bacon gently for 5-7 minutes, add onion and cook until golden. Add meat, fry for 3-5 minutes until brown.

Stir in sugar, pour over ale and lemon juice, add bay leaf, celery salt and seasoning.

Transfer to casserole dish and bake for 2 hours.

Serve with rice or mashed potato.

Sweet and sour turkey
2 Servings

1 large tomato
30g (1 oz) cucumber
1 small onion
½ small green pepper
2 tblsp vinegar
2 tblsp gluten free soy sauce
1 level tblsp brown sugar
¼ tsp cayenne powder (optional)
1 tblsp oil
1 clove garlic, crushed
350g (12 oz) cooked turkey, cubed
½ level tsp cornflour (cornstarch) or arrowroot
125g (4 oz) bean sprouts

Prepare vegetables and cut up. Mix vinegar, gluten free soy sauce, sugar and cayenne pepper.

Heat oil, fry garlic. Add turkey and fry 2 minutes. Add vegetables and fry a further 2 minutes.

Stir in the vinegar mixture, cover and cook for 2-3 minutes. Blend cornflour or arrowroot with water and stir into the sauce to thicken. Stir in bean sprouts and reheat.

Serve with rice noodles or rice.

CHECK ALL ingredient labels EVERY TIME YOU BUY

Somerset chicken in cider
4 Servings

8 chicken drumsticks
275ml (½ UK pint, 1¼ US cups) dry cider
2 level tsp French mustard
1 clove garlic, crushed
1 small onion, finely chopped
1 level tsp parsley
salt and pepper
1 level tblsp cornflour (cornstarch) or arrowroot

Preheat oven to 180°C (350°F, gas mark 4).

Put the drumsticks in a large casserole. Mix cider, mustard, garlic, onion, parsley and seasoning and pour over chicken. Cover and bake for 1 hour.

Remove chicken to serving dish. Mix cornflour or arrowroot with a little water to make a smooth cream, stir into the sauce and reheat on the hob if necessary, stirring until the mixture thickens evenly.

Spoon sauce over chicken or serve separately.

Spare ribs with cider
4-6 Servings

½ tsp dried sage
½ tsp mustard powder
½ tsp salt
½ tsp pepper
1.25 kg (2½ lb) spare rib of pork in one piece
2 eating apples, peeled and sliced
275ml (½ UK pint, 1¼ US cups) cider
275ml (½ UK pint, 1¼ US cups) stock

Preheat oven to 180°C (350°F, gas mark 4).

Mix sage, mustard, salt and pepper together and rub all over the meat.

Put apples, cider and stock into the bottom of a roasting tin. Stand meat on a rack over the apples. Bake for

CHECK ALL ingredient labels EVERY TIME YOU BUY

about 1¾ hours.

Cut the meat into individual ribs and serve with the apple sauce from the bottom of the tin.

Old fashioned spicy chicken
2 Servings

1 medium carrot, 1 small potato, 1 small leek, 1 chopped
   onion, 30g (1 oz) swede, ½ eating apple
2 cloves garlic
125g (4 oz) chicken
60ml (2 fl oz, ¼ US cup) oil
4 tsp medium curry powder
60g (2 oz) rice flour
1 large tomato or 2 tsp tomato purée
60g (2 oz) mushrooms
1 tblsp mango chutney
¼ tsp mixed herbs
½ tsp brown sugar
½ tsp Worcestershire sauce
salt and pepper
570ml (1 UK pint, 2½ US cups) chicken stock

Prepare and dice fruit and vegetables, crush garlic and chop, cut chicken into bite sized pieces.

Heat oil and add vegetables (except mushrooms and tomato), garlic and chicken (if raw). Stir fry for about 5 minutes.

Add curry powder and fry gently for a further 2 minutes. Add rice flour, beat in the stock with a whisk and continue stirring until it thickens.

Add tomato or tomato purée, mushrooms, apple, mango chutney, herbs, sugar, Worcestershire sauce, vanilla essence, salt and pepper . Stir gently. If using cooked chicken, add this now.

Cook gently for about half an hour. Serve with rice.

CHECK ALL ingredient labels EVERY TIME YOU BUY

Indian chicken with yogurt

4 Servings

4 chicken portions
570ml (1 pint, 2½ US cups) gluten free yogurt
1 garlic clove, crushed
1 level tsp ginger
1 medium onion, chopped
1 level tsp ground cumin
1 tblsp fresh coriander, chopped
3 green chillies (jalapenos)
2 tblsp tomato purée
salt

Preheat oven to 190°C (375°F, gas mark 5).

If you prefer a milder dish, remove seeds from chillies and discard. Chop chillies finely.

Lay the chicken portions in a casserole dish.

Mix remaining ingredients and pour over chicken. Cover and bake for 1 hour.

Serve hot with boiled rice.

Sozzled hearts

6 Servings

1.5kg (3 lb) lambs' or pigs' hearts
2 tblsp cider vinegar
275ml (½ UK pint, 1¼ US cups) stock
275ml (½ UK pint, 1¼ US cups) red wine
2 tblsp olive oil
salt and pepper
1 large onion, chopped
125g (4 oz) lean bacon, chopped
2 large potatoes, sliced
3 carrots, sliced
125g (4 oz) mushrooms, sliced

Prepare hearts and cut into cubes. Place in a flameproof casserole (one that will survive when heated on a ringof the stove) or a large saucepan, cover with stock, wine

CHECK ALL ingredient labels EVERY TIME YOU BUY

and olive oil. Add seasoning and onion. Marinate for 6 hours or overnight.

Add bacon to casserole, bring to the boil, cover and simmer for 15 minutes. Add carrots and potatoes, simmer for 25 minutes. Add mushrooms and simmer for a further 5 minutes. Check seasoning and serve.

Slow roast brisket of beef

6 Servings

1½ kg (3 lb) boned, rolled brisket of beef (unsalted)
500ml (1 pint, 2½ US cups) beef stock
1 bay leaf
3 cloves
black pepper

Put joint in baking tin and pour stock around. Add bay leaf, cloves, black pepper. Cover with foil or lid, bake at 220°C (425°F, gas mark 7) for 1 hour.

Reduce heat to 150°C (300°F, gas mark 2) and bake for 1 hour. Remove foil, turn oven back up to 220°C (425°F, gas mark 7) and cook for a further half an hour in the coolest part of the oven.

Remove joint from baking tin, strain the stock, taste and adjust seasoning, and serve as gravy. If you prefer a thicker gravy, heat in a pan and add half to one tablespoonful of rice flour, beating it in with a whisk and stirring continuously until thickened.

CHECK ALL ingredient labels EVERY TIME YOU BUY

Chicken pot pie

4 Servings

350g (12 oz) chicken, minced
1 small onion, finely chopped
4 rashers of lean bacon, chopped
250ml (8 fl oz, 1 US cup) of chicken stock or water
2 tblsp cooking sherry (optional)
1 tblsp cornflour (cornstarch) dissolved in a little water
700g potatoes (1½ lb), mashed with butter and milk
A little grated cheese (optional)

Preheat the oven to 220°C (425°F, gas mark 7).

Put the chicken, onion and bacon in a small saucepan with the stock and sherry, if used, and bring to the boil, breaking up the chicken as it heats. Reduce heat and simmer gently until cooked through (about 10 minutes).

Pour the cornflour and water mixture into the pan in a thin stream, stirring continuously. Bring back to the boil and stir until thickened.

Transfer the mix to a shallow ovenproof casserole or baking dish and top with mashed potatoes. If desired, sprinkle the top with a little grated cheese.

Bake in a hot oven until brown (about 30 minutes).

CHECK ALL ingredient labels EVERY TIME YOU BUY

RECIPES KIDS LOVE

Chicken and cashew nuts
8 Servings

8 large or 16 small mushrooms
1 tblsp oil
125g (4 oz) unsalted cashew nuts
6 water chestnuts, sliced
2 courgettes (zucchini), chopped
2 cloves garlic, crushed
2 chicken breasts, thinly sliced
1 carrot, peeled and thinly sliced
60g (2 oz) bamboo shoots, thinly sliced
3 tblsp water

If you can get dried Chinese mushrooms, these are the best. Alternatively, use straw mushrooms (available in tins from Chinese supermarkets), oyster mushrooms or ordinary mushrooms (in order of preference).

If using dried mushrooms, put them into cold water to cover and soak for 1 hour. Squeeze dry.

Slice mushrooms, removing hard parts, if present.

Sauté the nuts in the oil for 2 minutes, stirring continuously. Remove with a slotted spoon and drain on kitchen towel.

Sauté water chestnuts and courgettes for 1-2 minutes. Remove and set aside.

Sauté garlic and chicken for 2 minutes, turning frequently to ensure it is browned on all sides. Stir in mushrooms, carrot, bamboo shoots and reserved ingredients. Add water.

Cover and simmer for 3-5 minutes. Serve hot.

CHECK ALL ingredient labels EVERY TIME YOU BUY

Lasagne
4 Servings

1 packet gluten free lasagne
 or blanched white cabbage leaves
2 tblsp olive oil
2 onions, chopped
2 cloves garlic, crushed
500g minced beef
400g (14 oz) can tomatoes, chopped
1 gluten free beef or vegetable stock cube
1 tsp oregano
salt and pepper

Cheese sauce:
30g (1 oz) butter
30g (1 oz) rice flour
450ml (¾ UK pint, 1 US pint) milk
½ tsp salt
200g (7 oz) mature cheddar, grated by you*

Preheat oven to 180°C (350°F, gas mark 4).

If you haven't been able to get gluten free lasagne, take some leaves from a large white cabbage, keeping them whole, and immerse in boiling water for 2 or 3 minutes until they are soft and pliable. Drain.

Fry the onions and garlic gently in the olive oil until softened. Add the beef and break up, followed by the tomatoes and their juice, the stock cube, oregano and seasoning.

Bring to the boil and cook for about 10 minutes over a low heat, so it is just simmering.

Line the bottom of a lasagne dish with lasagne or cabbage leaves, cover with about half the meat and level off.

Add another layer of lasagne sheets or cabbage leaves. Cover with the rest of the meat and a final layer of lasagne/leaves.

In a small pan, melt the butter, stir in the milk and beat in the rice flour using a whisk. Keep stirring until it

CHECK ALL ingredient labels EVERY TIME YOU BUY

thickens. Check seasoning and add salt to taste. Bring to a full boil.

Remove from the heat, stir in half the cheese and when it has melted, pour over the mixture in the lasagne dish.

Sprinkle with the remaining cheese and transfer to the oven. Cook until brown and beautiful, and serve immediately.

* Don't buy ready grated cheese, unless you have checked that it has not been coated in "modified starch" or similar.

Barbecue-style spare ribs
4 Servings

4 spare rib chops
1 tblsp oil
salt and pepper
2 level tsp cornflour (cornstarch) or arrowroot
¼ tsp Worcestershire sauce
1 tsp yeast extract
1 tblsp vinegar
2 tblsp gluten free tomato ketchup
1 level tsp curry powder
1 level tblsp brown sugar

Brush chops with oil, season and grill on each side for about 7 minutes. Transfer to a casserole dish.

Preheat oven to 180°C (350°F, gas mark 4) .

Blend remaining ingredients together and heat in a small pan, stirring continuously until thickened.

Bake for 1 hour. Serve chops on a bed of rice, rice noodles, or mashed potato. Pour remaining sauce over, and add a serving of salad or sweetcorn on the side.

CHECK ALL ingredient labels EVERY TIME YOU BUY

Country lamb

6 Servings

2 kg (4 lb) shoulder of lamb
3 tblsp oil
150g (6 oz) onions, chopped
100g (4 oz) mushrooms, washed and sliced
400g (13½ oz) can peeled tomatoes
1 level tsp paprika
1 clove garlic crushed (optional)
1 sprig fresh or a pinch of dried rosemary
275ml (½ UK pint, 1¼ US cups) cider

Preheat oven to 180°C (350°F, gas mark 4).

Heat the oil in a large casserole of a type which will survive both on the hob and in the oven. Brown the lamb all over. Remove and set aside.

Fry onions until soft, add mushrooms, tomatoes, paprika, garlic, rosemary and cider. Check seasoning. Cook together for 6-7 minutes.

Return meat to pan. Cover casserole and bake for 2 hours. Remove cover and cook for a further 30 minutes.

Quick 'n easy spare ribs

2 or 3 spare ribs per person
1-2 tblsp gluten free soy sauce mixed with an equal
    quantity of oil

Brush the spare ribs with the mixture on both sides and put under a medium grill.

Grill for 10-15 minutes, brushing with further mixture frequently. Turn halfway through cooking.

Serve with egg fried rice or special fried rice. Also goes well with bean sprouts in soy sauce (Khang-namul) and/or vegetables in oyster sauce.

CHECK ALL ingredient labels EVERY TIME YOU BUY

Dutch chops
4 Servings

4 chump chops (sirloin) of lamb
4 slices Edam cheese
few spring (green) onions to garnish

Grill chops until virtually cooked, then top each one with a sprinkling of chopped spring (green) onions and a slice of cheese.

Grill for another minute or so until the cheese starts to melt and serve.

Devon hot pot
4 Servings

8 middle neck (shoulder) lamb chops
1 tblsp oil
1 large onion, finely chopped
500g (1 lb) potatoes, peeled and thickly sliced
2 tblsp chopped mint or mint jelly
2 level tsp brown sugar
1 level tsp salt, pepper
450ml (¾ UK pint, 1 US pint) chicken stock

Preheat oven to 180°C (350°F, gas mark 4).

Put a layer of potatoes in the bottom of a casserole dish, reserving 6 slices.

Fry chops in oil on both sides. Remove from pan, drain on kitchen towel and transfer to casserole dish.

Cover with onion, sprinkle with mint, half the sugar and seasoning. Add stock.

Arrange the reserved potato in the middle, brush with oil from the frying pan and sprinkle with the remaining sugar. Bake for 1½ hours.

CHECK ALL ingredient labels EVERY TIME YOU BUY

German stew

4 Servings

500g (1 lb) stewing beef, cubed
1 onion, chopped
2 carrots, peeled
2 sticks celery
4 tblsp fromage frais
2 level tsp cornflour (cornstarch) or arrowroot
2 level tsp chopped chives
salt and pepper

Cut the carrots into lengthwise strips, about 5cm x 1cm (2" by ½"). Cut celery into 5cm (2") lengths.

Put the meat and vegetables into a large pan or pressure cooker. Bring to the boil, cover and simmer for 1½ hours, or pressure cook on high for 20 minutes.

Mix the cornflour or arrowroot with a little water and stir in, stirring until thickened.

Stir in the chives and fromage frais. Check and adjust seasoning. Serve with sauerkraut (German pickled cabbage).

Jaffa chicken

4 Servings

4 chicken portions
salt and pepper
60g (2 oz) butter
2 large onions, finely chopped
1 tblsp cornflour (cornstarch)
275ml (½ UK pint, 1¼ US cups) chicken stock
½ level tsp thyme
½ level tsp rosemary
3 oranges

Preheat oven to 180°C (350°F, gas mark 4).

Skin chicken. Fry in butter until golden all over. Place in casserole dish. Fry onions until golden.

CHECK ALL ingredient labels EVERY TIME YOU BUY

Mix cornflour with a little of the stock to make a thin cream.

Remove from heat, blend in stock, cornflour mixture and herbs. Return to heat, stirring until sauce thickens.

Pour over chicken. Add grated rind and juice of 2 oranges.

Bake for 1 hour.

Finely slice the third orange, add to casserole and cook for a further 30 minutes.

Honey butter chicken
4 Servings

4 chicken portions
125g (4 oz) melted butter
2 tblsp cider vinegar
2 tblsp honey
1 garlic clove, crushed
2 level tsp salt
a pinch of marjoram
a pinch of dry mustard
black pepper
1 level tblsp chopped chives

Preheat oven to 200°C (400°F, gas mark 6).

Place the chicken portions in a single layer in a casserole dish.

Combine all the other ingredients except chives and mix well. Spoon over chicken and leave to marinate for 30 minutes.

Cover and bake for 15 minutes. Reduce heat to 170°C (325°F, gas mark 3) for 1 hour, or until tender.

Garnish with chives and serve.

CHECK ALL ingredient labels EVERY TIME YOU BUY

Pan pizza
2 Servings

1 cup gluten free flour (I used Doves Farm)
1 egg
a pinch of salt (optional)
one third cup of water (more or less as required)
Large can of tomatoes, puréed (add minced garlic and/or chilli/jalapeno if liked)
2-3 ounces grated cheese (whichever you like best)
Toppings: I used ham, cooked chicken and mushrooms

You need a frying pan with a tight fitting lid - glass for preference, so you can see what's happening.

Break egg into flour and salt, and knead together into rather sticky "breadcrumbs".

Add water, sufficient to make a sticky dough.

Break into 2 pieces for small pizzas, or leave whole.

Flour the worktop and flatten the dough into the size required to fit your pan. You will probably need to reflour a couple of times before you have finished this step.

Cook the first side until golden, turn over and add a layer of puréed tomato, cheese and other toppings. Pile them high, as they will shrink as they cook.

Put the lid on the pan and cook until the base is done, by which time the toppings will also be hot, and the cheese melted.

Serve immediately.

Savory pancakes
3 Servings (3 pancakes each)

275ml (½ UK pint, 1¼ US cups) milk
1-2 eggs
a pinch of salt
115g (3½ oz) rice flour
Oil to fry

CHECK ALL ingredient labels EVERY TIME YOU BUY

Suggested fillings:
Grated cheese — Tuna mayonnaise — Chicken and bacon
Cheese and crispy bacon — Chicken and mushroom
Bacon and tomatoes

Put the milk and eggs with the salt into a large jug and beat to break up the eggs. Sprinkle on the rice flour and mix in with a whisk, one tablespoonful at a time. Leave to stand for about 10 minutes, then stir again with the whisk so that the flour is evenly distributed (and not in a sticky mass at the bottom).

Using a small frying pan about the size of the pancakes you want (about 20cm diameter), heat a very small amount of oil to coat the base completely. Pour off excess oil into a saucer.

Pour a small quantity of the batter into the pan, about half as much as it seems you need. Tip the pan to coat the base evenly. Cook for a minute or so until little holes appear all over and the edges turn brown and start to curl up.

Using a palette knife, loosen the edges of the pancake and flip it over to cook the other side. Turn out onto a plate and cover with a clean dry cloth to keep warm.

Add a little more oil and tip out as before (you can use the oil from the saucer if there is enough). Pour in a similar amount of batter and repeat the process as described, stacking the pancakes on top of each other on the plate and covering with the cloth.

When all the pancakes are cooked, put one at a time onto a plate, add the filling at one end or spread thinly on one side and roll up, then transfer to a plate for serving.

CHECK ALL ingredient labels EVERY TIME YOU BUY

Quick chicken risotto

4-6 Servings

250g (½ lb) cooked chicken
2 cups brown rice and 4 cups water
 or 2 cups white rice and 2 cups water
60g (2 oz) chopped mushrooms
150g (5 oz) mixed diced vegetables
2 cloves of garlic, finely chopped
gluten free chicken stock cube
salt and pepper

Put all the ingredients together in a saucepan.

Bring to the boil and stir once, cover and turn heat down very low.

Continue to cook until the liquid is absorbed and the rice is light and fluffy.

DO NOT STIR DURING COOKING. If you need to check how much water is left, carefully push the rice aside with a fork.

Sweet sour pork, Hong Kong style

4 Servings

750g (1½ lb) lean pork, cubed
125g (4 oz) cornflour (cornstarch)
½ level tsp gluten free baking powder
a pinch of salt
150ml (¼ UK pint, $\frac{5}{8}$ US cup) milk
oil for deep frying
570ml (1 UK pint, 2½ US cups) GF sweet and sour sauce

Sieve 100g (3 oz) cornflour, baking powder and salt. Mix with milk to make a thin batter.

Heat oil. Coat the pork cubes in the remaining cornflour, dip in the batter and deep fry.

Serve with sweet sour sauce and rice or noodles. Best with other dishes as part of a Chinese meal.

CHECK ALL ingredient labels EVERY TIME YOU BUY

Roast chicken

1-8 Servings

500g (1¼ lb) bird (Poussin) – 1 serving
1 kg (2½ lb) bird (Spring chicken) – 2-3 servings
1.5-2 kg (3-4 lb) bird – 4 servings
2-3 kg (4-6 lb) bird – 8 servings

Remove the little pads of fat just inside the cavity and put to one side. Stuff and weigh bird to calculate cooking time. Place on a rack, in a roasting tin, tie feet together and cover the ends with the fat set aside. Sprinkle the bird with salt.

Surround smaller birds with potatoes and drizzle with oil, or for larger ones add potatoes partway through roasting. **NOTE**: Potatoes will need at least 80 minutes to roast properly (you can speed this up by deep-frying them for a few minutes before putting them in, in which case don't add any more oil - or you could put the potatoes in first, and add the bird when they are half cooked).

Roast Poussin for 40-45 minutes at 190°C (375°F, gas mark 5), Spring chicken for 50-60 minutes at the same temperature, others for 45 minutes a kilo (20 minutes a pound) plus 20 minutes at 200°C (400°F, gas mark 6).

Remove chicken from rack and tip the juices inside into a small saucepan. Put on a serving dish and surround with the potatoes from the roasting pan. Leave to rest while you make the gravy.

Use a stuffing based on rice or serve extra vegetables. Traditional accompaniments are bacon rolls, chipolatas and gravy. I generally serve with green beans or runner beans stringed and snapped into pieces about 5cm (2") long (small green beans can be left whole).

CHECK ALL ingredient labels EVERY TIME YOU BUY

Sweet and sour meatballs
4 Servings

Meatballs:
450g (1 lb) minced beef
1 tsp salt
ground black pepper to taste
¼ tsp Chinese five spice powder
2 cloves garlic, crushed
2 tblsp cornflour (cornstarch) or rice flour
oil to fry

Sauce:
a handful of fresh needle beans
1 red pepper
1-2 carrots
1 onion
1-2 courgettes (zucchini)
1 slice root ginger
1 small tin of pineapple in juice
275ml (½ UK pint, 1¼ US cups) chicken stock or water
75ml (3 fl oz, $\frac{1}{3}$ US cup) white wine vinegar or cider
    vinegar
1 tblsp gluten free soy sauce
1 tblsp brown sugar
1 tblsp cornflour (cornstarch)

Mix the beef with the garlic and seasonings. Shape into 2-3cm (1") balls.

Roll in the flour and fry gently in hot oil for 5 to 10 minutes.

Remove and keep hot.

Top and tail the beans and cook in boiling salted water for about 5 minutes.

De-seed the red pepper and cut into large strips. Peel carrots and cut into thin diagonal slices. Peel onion and slice into wedges. Top and tail courgettes and slice thinly. Peel and finely chop the ginger. Chop the

CHECK ALL ingredient labels EVERY TIME YOU BUY

pineapple into small pieces, retaining the juice.

Mix soy sauce, brown sugar, cornflour and vinegar together.

Heat oil and stir fry vegetables and ginger for a minute or two, then add stock or water and simmer briefly until the vegetables are just cooked, but still slightly crisp.

Add vinegar mix and the pineapple with its juice, stirring continuously.

Heat to thicken, add meatballs and warm though.

Serve with rice or rice noodles.

Barbecue-style chicken drumsticks
2-3 Servings

6 chicken drumsticks, skin on
1 tblsp oil
2 tsp Worcestershire sauce
2 tsp caster sugar
4 tsp cider vinegar
3 tsp gluten free tomato ketchup
a pinch of garlic powder

Mix all ingredients except chicken together. Brush drumsticks with the mixture and put under a medium grill for about 15 minutes, turning 2 or 3 times during cooking and brushing with the barbecue mixture frequently.

Goes well with sauté potatoes or rösti and sweetcorn or peas, with chunky tomato salad on the side.

CHECK ALL ingredient labels EVERY TIME YOU BUY

MAIN COURSES: FISH BASED

Cod fiesta
6 Servings

15g (½ oz) butter
125g (4 oz) green or red peppers, chopped
125g (4 oz) mushrooms, chopped
a pinch of mace or nutmeg
6 x 150g (5 oz) cod steaks, fresh or frozen
60g (2 oz) cheddar, finely grated
¼ tsp paprika
salt and pepper to taste

Preheat grill.

Melt butter, add peppers and mushrooms and cook gently for about 10 minutes. Add seasoning and mace or nutmeg.

Place cod steaks in grill pan, grill on medium heat for 5 minutes on each side (10 minutes for frozen cod steaks).

Spoon pepper mixture on top of each steak, sprinkle with grated cheese and put back under the grill for a further 5 minutes until the cheese is bubbling and golden.

Serve with green vegetables or salad.

Poached trout
4 Servings

4x250g (8 oz) rainbow trout, cleaned
4 stuffed green olives, cut in half
3 bay leaves, 2 sprigs parsley
1 small onion, quartered
4 strips lemon rind
4 cloves

Put the bay leaves, onion, lemon rind, parsley and cloves into a litre (2 pints) of water and bring to the boil.
Simmer for 5 minutes. Strain into a large shallow pan or fish kettle.

CHECK ALL ingredient labels EVERY TIME YOU BUY

Place the washed trout into the pan, cover with lid and bring slowly back to the boil. Reduce heat and simmer for 10 minutes.

Remove from heat and allow to cool in the liquid. When cool, lift out and drain.

Place each trout on a serving dish, with a slice of olive over each eye. Serve chilled.

Mackerel casserole
4 Servings

4 filleted mackerel
1 garlic clove, crushed
125g (4 oz) mushrooms, chopped
100g (3 oz) sweetcorn
100g (3 oz) peas
1 large onion, chopped
400ml (13½ oz) can chopped tomatoes
½ tsp dried fennel
1 tblsp fresh parsley, chopped
salt and pepper

Preheat oven to 180°C (350°F, gas mark 4).

Cut mackerel into 2-3cm (1") wide strips, and place in a casserole dish. Add garlic and vegetables. Mix tomatoes with fennel, parsley and seasoning. Add to casserole, stirring to mix.

Cover and bake for 1 hour.

CHECK ALL ingredient labels EVERY TIME YOU BUY

RECIPES KIDS LOVE

Sweet and sour fish

8 Servings

2 kg (4 lb) fresh whole bream, mullet or bass
3 cloves garlic, sliced
8 slices fresh root ginger
2 tblsp gluten free soy sauce
1 tblsp rice wine or dry sherry (optional)
3 large or 6 small mushrooms
2 spring (green) onions
125g (4 oz) bamboo shoots
1 carrot
1 tblsp peas, fresh or frozen
60g (2 oz) cornflour (cornstarch)
oil for frying
570ml (1 UK pint, 2½ US cups) gluten free sweet and
   sour sauce

If you can get dried Chinese mushrooms, these are the best. Alternatively, use straw mushrooms (available in tins from Chinese supermarkets), oyster mushrooms or ordinary mushrooms (in order of preference).

If using dried mushrooms, put them into cold water to cover and soak for 1 hour. Squeeze dry.

Clean fish, scraping off the scales with sharp knife. Rinse well.

Make diagonal slits into the flesh on both sides of fish, insert garlic and half of the ginger into the slits.

Place fish in dish and pour over soy sauce and rice wine or sherry. Leave to marinade for at least 30 minutes.

Pat fish dry and coat with cornflour. Heat oil until very hot and fry fish on both sides until crisp, about 4 minutes. Drain on kitchen towel and transfer to serving dish.

CHECK ALL ingredient labels EVERY TIME YOU BUY

Chop vegetables and remaining ginger.

Reheat sweet sour sauce in a pan, add vegetables and cook for a further 2 minutes. Pour over fish and serve immediately.

Cheese plaice
1 Serving

1 fillet of plaice
butter
salt and pepper
60g (2 oz) grated cheese

Preheat oven to 175°C (Gas mark 4, 350°F).

Dot fillet with butter, season, sprinkle with cheese and bake for 20 minutes.

CHECK ALL ingredient labels EVERY TIME YOU BUY

MAIN COURSES: VEGETABLE BASED

Song-i-pahb
(Korean rice and mushrooms)
2-4 Servings

2 cups brown rice and 4 cups water
 or 2 cups white rice and 2 cups water
1 cup mushrooms
2-3 crushed cloves garlic
2-3 sliced onions
2 tblsp dark gluten free soy sauce
1 tblsp sesame oil
1 tblsp Kaey-Garu or sesame seeds
1 tsp salt
pepper

Wash rice and drain.

Mix mushrooms, onions, garlic, gluten free soy sauce, oil and sesame seeds, salt and pepper. Fry mixture for 2 minutes in a large pan.

Add rice and water and stir. Cover tightly and bring to the boil.

Reduce heat to lowest and cook for about 30 minutes until rice is dry and fluffy.

When cooked, turn onto a hot platter and serve at once.

Alternatively, using a metal casserole dish instead of a pan, the dish can be transferred to a fairly hot oven once it has come to the boil and served from the cooking dish.

Variation:

Add 2 cups of sliced vegetables to taste, eg. carrots, courgettes (zucchini), diced potato, leeks etc. with the rice.

CHECK ALL ingredient labels EVERY TIME YOU BUY

Frittata (Italian omelette)
6-8 Servings

250g (8 oz) courgettes (zucchini)
1 red onion
1 green pepper
6 cherry tomatoes
6 free range eggs
Salt and pepper
90g (3 oz) grated cheese
Butter or olive oil

Core green pepper and slice finely. Peel and slice onion finely. Clean courgettes and slice thinly. Quarter tomatoes.

In the omelette pan, heat oil or butter and add prepared vegetables. Sauté gently together until softened.

Beat eggs with salt and freshly ground black pepper. Pour over vegetables and stir in cheese.

As the egg cooks, loosen the sides and allow the uncooked part to flow to the bottom of the pan, then lower heat and cover pan with lid.

After 10 minutes remove lid and slide pan under grill to brown.

Loosen sides and turn out onto plate. Cut into wedges to eat hot or cold with salad.

Cottage cheese casserole
4 Servings

3 eggs, lightly beaten
725ml (1¼ UK pints, 3¼ US cups) cottage cheese
1 small diced onion
salt and black pepper to taste

Preheat oven to 180°C (350°F, gas mark 4).

Mix all ingredients and pour into a casserole dish. Bake for 45-50 minutes, or until it is firm and pulls away from the sides of the pan. Serve warm.

CHECK ALL ingredient labels EVERY TIME YOU BUY

Nut croquettes
4 Servings

750g (1½ lb) boiled potatoes
25g (1 oz) butter
125g (4 oz) broken walnuts
1 level tsp curry powder
1 egg, beaten
1 heaped tblsp dried milk
50g (2 oz) desiccated coconut
Little vegetable oil
Few lemon slices
Few sprigs of cress

Mash potatoes and combine with the butter, walnuts, curry powder, egg and milk. Beat well with a wooden spoon to make a smooth mixture, adding fresh milk as needed - the mixture should be stiff enough to handle.

Cool. Divide into eight portions, and roll each in coconut. Shape into rectangular shapes about 1 cm (½") thick.

Fry gently in hot oil, browning both sides. Drain.

Serve croquettes piled on a hot dish, garnished with lemon slices and sprigs of cress.

Khichri (Indian lentil and rice kedgeree)
4-6 Servings

2 cups brown rice and 5 cups water
 or 2 cups white rice and 3 cups water
1 cup red lentils
2 cardamoms
2 cloves
60g (1 oz) ghee or butter
1 chopped onion
1 inch piece cinnamon
¼ tsp whole cumin seeds
1 tsp turmeric
salt and pepper

Wash and soak rice and lentils separately in plenty of water for half an hour. Drain well.

CHECK ALL ingredient labels EVERY TIME YOU BUY

Fry half the onion in the butter. Remove onion and set aside for use as garnish.

Remove seeds from cardamom pods and crush with cloves, discarding pods.

Add spices, salt and pepper to the pan and cook for 2 minutes. Add remaining onion and cook until brown.

Add lentils to onions and spices in pan and stir. Add rice, stir again and cook until rice begins to stick to the bottom of the pan. Add the measured water and bring to the boil.

Cover and cook over a low heat until rice and lentils are both cooked and water has been absorbed.

Garnish with reserved onions and serve.

Nut roast
4-6 Servings

25g (1 oz, 2 tblsp) butter
1 small onion
1 small carrot
1 stalk celery
1 tblsp tomato purée/paste
225g (8 oz, 1 US cup) skinned and chopped tomatoes
2 eggs
1 tblsp chopped parsley
salt and freshly ground black pepper
225g (8 oz, 2 US cups) finely chopped nuts

Preheat oven to 230°C (450°F, gas mark 8).

Prepare and chop onion, carrot and celery.

Melt the butter in a pan; add the vegetables and cook until softened. Add the tomatoes and tomato purée and cook for 5 minutes.

Beat eggs well with parsley and salt and pepper to taste.Stir in the nuts and vegetables.

Transfer to a greased loaf tin or ovenproof dish and bake for 30-35 minutes.

Turn out and serve hot with vegetables and gravy, or cold with salad.

CHECK ALL ingredient labels EVERY TIME YOU BUY

RECIPES KIDS LOVE

Cheesy stuffed marrow
2 Servings

4 slices vegetable marrow* about 2-3cm (1-1½") thick
30g (1 oz) mushrooms
2 medium tomatoes
120g (4 oz) strong grated cheese
1 medium onion
2-3 potatoes
few drops Worcestershire sauce
salt and pepper
small pinch dry mustard
pinch sugar (optional)
oil

Preheat oven to 220°C (425°F, gas mark 7).

Peel and de-seed marrow. Put the slices into an ovenproof dish and add about 250ml of salted water. Bake for about 25 minutes. Carefully pour off any excess water. Leave the oven on.

Peel potatoes and cook in boiling salted water.

Chop mushrooms, leeks and onions and mix together, heat a very little oil and cook gently for a few minutes until soft. Mix in a large bowl with the cheese, Worcestershire sauce and mustard.

Mash potatoes and add to the bowl, mixing well. Adjust seasoning and stuff marrow slices with the mixture.

Cut tomatoes in half and put one half on each marrow slice, season and bake for a further 20 minutes.

* Vegetable marrow is a winter squash that looks like an overgrown zucchini.

CHECK ALL ingredient labels EVERY TIME YOU BUY

MAIN COURSE ACCOMPANIMENTS: SIDE DISHES

Nasi Goreng (Spicy fried rice)

3-4 Servings

2 eggs
60g (2 oz) meat or chicken, raw or cooked
a handful of cooked peeled prawns (optional)
6 mange tout pea pods
6 baby sweetcorn
1 cup cooked rice
1-2 cloves of garlic
2 spring (green) onions
1-2 small green chillies (jalapenos) (optional)
1-2 tblsp gluten free soy sauce
oil for frying

If using raw meat, cut into small pieces and fry gently in the oil until well cooked but not browned. Remove from pan.

Cut pre-cooked meat into 1cm (½") cubes. Cut the pea pods and baby sweetcorn into 5-6 pieces. Chop chilli very finely (discard seeds if you prefer).

Heat oil in a wok or other large frying pan and pour in eggs, cook until set, turn over to set the other side, then remove from pan and chop.

Put the spring (green) onions, garlic and all dry ingredients except the egg and rice into the wok. Stir fry for 2-3 minutes. Add the rice to the pan and stir fry until the rice is well heated through.

Put the chopped egg back into the pan along with the soy sauce.

Continue to cook, stirring to distribute the soy sauce evenly. Serve immediately.

CHECK ALL ingredient labels EVERY TIME YOU BUY

Dahi (Indian curd/yogurt)
Makes 600ml

570ml (1 UK pint, 2½ US cups) full cream milk
juice of 1 lime or ½ lemon

Bring milk to blood heat, add lemon or lime juice and stir well. Leave covered in a warm place for 12-15 hours until set.

To make a new batch, reserve a tablespoon of the previous batch and use this instead of the citrus juice.

Raita (Indian spiced curd)
Makes 1-2 cups

1-2 cups dahi or plain gluten free yogurt
chopped coriander
salt and pepper
a pinch of dry mustard
choice of vegetables (see below)
finely chopped garlic (optional)

Press out dahi and let excess water drip out. Season with other ingredients, then mix with any of the following:
Skinned and chopped tomatoes
Grated raw carrot
Peeled and finely cut cucumber
Cooked sliced potatoes and chopped chives

Serve chilled as a side dish to go with curry or Tandoori.

Kaey-garu (toasted sesame seeds)
As required

Cook sesame seeds in a thick frying pan without fat over a low heat, stirring all the time. When just browned take from the heat and crush. They will smell beautifully fragrant. Use as a garnish or for flavoring.

CHECK ALL ingredient labels EVERY TIME YOU BUY

Pulao (Pakistani pilau rice)
2-4 Servings

2 cups brown rice and 4 cups boiling water
 or 2 cups white rice and 2 cups boiling water
2 tblsp oil
salt and pepper
yellow food die (optional)

Fry rice gently in the oil, stirring all the time. Add plenty of salt and pepper, and when the rice begins to look translucent, slowly add the liquid.

When all the water has been added, stir, cover and cook over a very low heat until all the water has been absorbed.

Sprinkle several drops of food die over the cooked rice, and serve.

Dahl (Indian lentils)
4-6 Servings

250g (8 oz) red lentils
570ml (1 UK pint, 2½ US cups) water
1 small piece ginger root, peeled and chopped finely
 or 2 tsp Punjabi spice mixture
salt and pepper
2 tsp ghee or butter
1 onion, thinly sliced into rings

Wash lentils and cook in water with the ginger or spice mix, salt and pepper until soft.

Beat with an eggbeater until reasonably smooth. Put into a serving dish.

Fry the onion rings in the ghee or butter until brown, pour over lentils and serve. (This is the authentic recipe used by a friend of mine. However, I find the onion is much better drained and used without the frying fat.)

CHECK ALL ingredient labels EVERY TIME YOU BUY

RECIPES KIDS LOVE

Egg fried rice
2-3 Servings

2 eggs
1 cup cooked rice
1-2 cloves of garlic
2 spring (green) onions
1 tblsp gluten free soy sauce
oil for frying

Chop spring (green) onions, crush and chop garlic finely. Beat eggs lightly. Heat oil and pour in eggs, cook until set, turn over to set the other side, then remove from pan and chop.

Put the spring onions, garlic and rice into the pan and fry until popping slightly. Stir and continue to cook until all the rice is well heated on all sides.

Return egg to pan, pour over soy sauce, stirring to distribute the soy sauce evenly. Serve immediately.

Potato latkes
2-3 Servings

Half an onion, chopped finely
1 large potato, peeled and chopped finely
1 small can sweetcorn, drained (optional)
2 tblsp rice flour
2 tblsp chopped parsley
2 eggs, beaten
Salt and pepper
5 tblsp dried milk powder
Oil for frying

Mix all ingredients except oil together and fry like pancakes in hot oil. Brown both sides well and drain on kitchen towel before serving.

CHECK ALL ingredient labels EVERY TIME YOU BUY

MAIN COURSE ACCOMPANIMENTS: SAUCES

Cho-jang (Korean soy and vinegar sauce)
Makes 600 ml

275ml (½ UK pint, 1¼ US cups) good quality vinegar
275ml (½ UK pint, 1¼ US cups) gluten free soy sauce
90g (3 oz) brown sugar
pine nuts to taste
finely chopped onions (optional)
crushed sesame seeds (optional)

Dissolve the sugar in the liquid ingredients and add pine nuts to taste. Finely chopped onion or crushed sesame seeds may be added if liked. Use as a fish dip.

Savory butters
Makes 125g

125g (4 oz) butter

Maitre d'Hotel butter
2 tblsp chopped parsley
1 tblsp lemon juice

Mustard butter
1 tblsp dry mustard
¼ tsp lemon juice

Curry butter
1 tsp curry powder
1 tblsp lemon juice

Tomato butter
2 level tblsp tomato purée
¼ tsp lemon juice

Cream the butter, then beat in the other ingredients.

Form into a roll the diameter of the pat you wish to serve. Wrap in greaseproof paper and refrigerate.

To serve, just unwrap and slice off the number of pats required.

CHECK ALL ingredient labels EVERY TIME YOU BUY

Traditional horseradish sauce
Makes 250 ml

2 tblsp wine vinegar
2 tsp dry mustard
salt and pepper
180g (6 oz) fresh horseradish
275ml (½ UK pint, 1¼ US cups) double (heavy) cream

This is best made fresh at the time it is to be served and is *extremely* pungent.

Grate the horseradish into a small basin and combine with the vinegar, mustard and seasoning.

Stiffly whip the cream and fold into the mixture.

Check seasoning, transfer to a sauce boat, and serve.

Gravy for roast chicken
juices from inside chicken and from roasting tin
1-2 tblsp rice flour
1 or 2 gluten free chicken stock cubes
a pinch of rosemary or your favourite herb for chicken
boiling water to make up quantity required

Drain off as much fat from the roasting tin as you can, pouring it into a bowl or other heatproof container.

Pour the remaining juices into a small saucepan with the juices from inside the chicken.

Add the rice flour and beat with a whisk until completely dissolved. Add the stock cube and put the kettle on.

Stir over the heat continuously, addingthe herbs and boiling water. Keep stirring until the stock cube dissolves and the mixture thickens. Taste and adjust seasoning. Serve.

CHECK ALL ingredient labels EVERY TIME YOU BUY

Mint sauce
Makes 300ml

8 tblsp mint leaves
2 level tblsp caster sugar
150ml (¼ UK pint, ⅝ US cup) boiling water
150ml (¼ UK pint, ⅝ US cup) wine vinegar

Put the mint leaves on a chopping board and sprinkle with sugar. Chop finely.

Put into a bowl, add the boiling water and vinegar. Mix well and leave to stand in a warm place for 30 minutes, then transfer to a serving jug.

Sweet and sour sauce with pineapple
6-8 Servings

1 clove garlic, crushed
250g (8 oz) can pineapple
2 level tblsp caster sugar
4 tblsp cider vinegar
4 tblsp gluten free soy sauce
2 level tblsp cornflour (cornstarch)

Fry garlic in a little oil and drain on kitchen paper.

Drain pineapple, reserving juice. Cut fruit into chunks and put in a pan over a medium heat with garlic, sugar, vinegar and gluten free soy sauce.

Make juice up to 200ml (½ pint) with water. Use a little of this to blend with the cornflour to make a smooth paste. Stir into pan along with the remaining juice and water.

Bring to the boil, stirring continuously. The liquid will start to thicken and change color, becoming translucent when completely cooked.

Season to taste and serve hot.

CHECK ALL ingredient labels EVERY TIME YOU BUY

RECIPES KIDS LOVE

Hot tomato sauce
4 Servings

1 kg (2 lb) fresh tomatoes, skinned
1 medium onion, sliced
30g (1 oz) butter
1 level tblsp olive oil
2 cloves garlic, crushed
2 level tsp fresh basil
1 bay leaf
2 level tsp fresh rosemary
1 level tsp fresh parsley
150ml (¼ UK pint, ⅝ US cup) stock
salt and black pepper
1 level tblsp tomato purée

Put all the ingredients into a large saucepan and season to taste.

Cover and simmer for about 30 minutes.

Blend until smooth. Return to pan and reheat.

Barbecue sauce
6-8 Servings

2 tblsp Worcestershire sauce
2 tblsp caster sugar
4 tblsp red wine vinegar
3 tblsp gluten free tomato ketchup
2 tblsp gluten free soy sauce
2 cloves garlic, crushed
2 bay leaves
few drops Tabasco sauce

Mix all ingredients, stirring until sugar is dissolved. Allow to stand overnight.

CHECK ALL ingredient labels EVERY TIME YOU BUY

Apple sauce
6-8 Servings

500g (1 lb) cooking apples, peeled, cored and sliced
3 tblsp water
2 tblsp lemon juice
30g (1 oz) butter
2 level tblsp sugar

Put apples into a pan with the water and lemon juice. Cover and cook gently for 10 minutes, stirring occasionally until the apples are soft.

Beat well and stir in butter. Add sugar to taste. Serve hot or cold.

Salsa
4 Servings

1 large can peeled tomatoes
1 small bunch fresh coriander
1 medium/large onion
1 clove garlic
salt

Roughly chop all ingredients and process in a blender. Season to taste. Serve chilled.

Cranberry sauce
6-8 Servings

500g (1 lb) cranberries
180g (6 oz) caster sugar
150ml (¼ UK pint, $\frac{5}{8}$ US cup) water

Put all the ingredients into a saucepan, cover and simmer for about 15 minutes until cranberries are tender. Turn into a serving dish and allow to cool.

CHECK ALL ingredient labels EVERY TIME YOU BUY

Classic sweet and sour sauce

Makes 500 ml

2 tblsp cornflour (cornstarch) or arrowroot
2 tblsp cider vinegar
2 tblsp gluten free soy sauce
2 tblsp dark brown sugar
450ml (¾ UK pint, 1 US pint) water
1 medium carrot (optional)

Mix cornflour to a thin paste with the water, add vinegar, soy sauce and sugar.

Put into a pan, cook and stir continuously over a low heat until the mixture boils and becomes thickened and translucent.

Cut the carrot into very fine julienne strips and stir into the sauce just before serving.

CHECK ALL ingredient labels EVERY TIME YOU BUY

VEGETABLE DISHES

Patate alla Poppea
4 Servings

30g (1 oz) butter
1 kg (2¼ lb) potatoes
275ml (½ UK pint, 1¼ US cups) milk
salt and pepper
¼ tsp nutmeg
1 level tblsp fresh parsley, chopped

Preheat oven to 200°C (400°F, gas mark 6).

Butter a deep pie dish.

Peel and chop potatoes in chunks. Pile into dish and pour over milk. Add seasoning and nutmeg.

Bake uncovered for 45 minutes.

Brussels sprouts with chestnuts
6 Servings

180g (6 oz) chestnuts, fresh or canned
275ml (½ UK pint, 1¼ US cups) stock
500g (1 lb) Brussels sprouts
60g (1 oz) butter

Peel fresh chestnuts, or drain canned ones. Simmer in stock for 30 minutes. Drain.

Prepare Brussels sprouts and cook. Drain.

Melt butter in a pan and add Brussels sprouts and chestnuts. Heat gently for 3-5 minutes, shaking well until heated through and well coated.

Serve.

Goes well with turkey, pheasant or beef.

CHECK ALL ingredient labels EVERY TIME YOU BUY

Courgettes à la Grecque
6 Servings

500g (1 lb) courgettes (zucchini), sliced
1 tsp salt
3 tblsp olive oil
juice of half a lemon
275ml (½ UK pint, 1¼ US cups) water
1 bay leaf
1 sprig thyme
6 black peppercorns, crushed
6 coriander seeds, crushed
3 tomatoes, skinned and chopped
1 clove garlic, crushed

Place all ingredients in a heavy saucepan. Bring to the boil, cover and turn the heat right down.

Cook for 25 minutes, cool and drain. Remove herbs. Arrange in a dish and chill.

Khang-namul
(Korean bean sprouts in soy sauce)
4-6 Servings

1 kg (2 lb) bean sprouts
sesame oil
1 tblsp gluten free dark soy sauce
1 tblsp toasted sesame seeds
2 chopped spring (green) onions
pepper

Cook bean sprouts until tender in boiling water. Drain and stir a little sesame oil into the sprouts, then add soy sauce, sesame seeds, onions and pepper.

Continue cooking very gently until all the seasonings have been absorbed.

CHECK ALL ingredient labels EVERY TIME YOU BUY

Taung-bho-hmo
(Burmese spiced mushrooms)
2 Servings

2 large onions
4 cloves garlic
2 strips lemon peel
500g (1 lb) mushrooms
4 tblsp oil
1 tsp turmeric
salt
1 tblsp lemon juice

Chop one of the onions, the garlic, and the lemon peel. Put into a blender and blend together, or chop very finely and mix together.

Clean and thickly slice mushrooms, discarding stems. Slice the other onion.

Heat oil and add turmeric, salt, mixed ingredients and the sliced onion. Cook for a few minutes, add mushrooms, stir and cook over a low heat until tender.

Sprinkle with lemon juice just before serving. Serve with boiled rice or a plain pilau.

Runner beans with garlic
6 Servings

500g (1 lb) runner beans, cut into chunks, NOT sliced
60g (2 oz) butter
1 clove garlic
1 level tblsp chopped parsley

Cook fresh beans in boiling salted water for 10 minutes. Drain.

Heat butter in pan, add crushed garlic and parsley. Stir in beans and cook together gently for 3 minutes.

CHECK ALL ingredient labels EVERY TIME YOU BUY

Peas with lettuce
6-8 Servings

About 10 lettuce leaves
750g (1½ lb) shelled or frozen peas
1 level tsp mint, chopped (optional)
1½ tblsp butter
salt and pepper

Wash the lettuce leaves and use half to line a large saucepan.

Put in the peas, sprinkle with the mint, if used, and the butter cut into small pieces.

Cover with remaining lettuce. Put lid on pan, and cook on low heat for 20 minutes, shaking now and then to prevent the peas from sticking.

Season, turn into a warmed serving dish. Serve hot.

Zesty red cabbage
4 Servings

500g (1 lb) red cabbage
60g (2 oz) butter
4 cloves
1 tblsp vinegar
60g (2 oz) sultanas
2 level tblsp brown sugar
salt and black pepper

Preheat oven to 170°C (350°F, gas mark 4).

Shred cabbage, wash and drain.

Melt butter in pan, add cabbage, cloves, vinegar, sultanas, sugar, salt and pepper. Stir to mix.

Cover pan. Bake in the coolest part of the oven for 2 hours until tender.

CHECK ALL ingredient labels EVERY TIME YOU BUY

Pisellini alla Capricciosa (Peas with ham)

4 Servings

350g (12 oz) peas, fresh or frozen
60g (2 oz) butter
1 small onion, diced
half a red pepper, diced
60g (2 oz) ham diced

Cook peas.

Meanwhile, fry onions in butter for 5-7 minutes until golden. Add red pepper and ham and cook for a further 3 minutes.

Drain the peas. Combine with onions, pepper and ham. Check seasoning and serve in a warmed serving dish.

Mixed vegetables with oyster sauce

8 Servings

1 small turnip, peeled
2 large carrots, scrubbed
half a red pepper, de-seeded
half a green pepper, de-seeded
1 large or 2 small courgettes (zucchini), peeled
2 tblsp oil
125g (4 oz) mushrooms
2 tblsp gluten free oyster sauce
6 tblsp water

Dice turnip and carrots. Chop peppers and courgettes. Break cauliflower into small florets. Slice large mushrooms or remove and chop stalks of button mushrooms.

Sauté peppers, courgettes and mushrooms for 1-2 minutes. Remove from pan and set aside.

Sauté carrots and turnip for 1-2 minutes. Add water and oyster sauce. Cover and cook for 4-5 minutes.

Add reserved vegetables, turn up the heat and cook for a further 2-3 minutes. Vegetables should be cooked, but remain crisp.

CHECK ALL ingredient labels EVERY TIME YOU BUY

RECIPES KIDS LOVE

Rösti (Swiss potato pancakes)
2-4 Servings

1kg (2 lbs) cold boiled potatoes
1 large onion, finely chopped (optional)
1 clove garlic, crushed and finely chopped (optional)
(60g) 2 oz butter or 4 tblsp olive oil or a mixture
1 tsp salt
2 tblsp milk

This is a very variable recipe, each family having their own favourite way of making it.

Note: Onions and garlic are not part of the "classic" rösti - about 30% of recipes include one or other (more often onions than garlic).

It is important that the potatoes be cooked at least 1 day beforehand. Boil them unpeeled until semi-tender the day before preparation.

Peel and grate the potatoes.

Heat butter or oil in skillet. If using onions or garlic, cook very gently until soft. Add potatoes and stir into the onions or garlic, sprinkle with salt. Using a spatula, press together to form a round loaf or patty. Sprinkle with milk and **cover tightly**. Reduce heat as soon as the potatoes begin to sizzle.

Fry very slowly for another 30 minutes. Do not stir.

During this time, a brown crust will form on the bottom.

Cover pan with a hot platter and flip the Rösti onto it.

Serve as a meal accompaniment or as a base for things normally served on toast, for example fried eggs, cheese or baked beans.

CHECK ALL ingredient labels EVERY TIME YOU BUY

Rösti variations

Rösti is generally only cooked on one side, and then served with that side uppermost. However, some recipes say to flip the rösti halfway through cooking and brown the other side. This would probably be the best way to cook them to use as a toast substitute, or you could just use them the wrong way up (without flipping).

Bernese Rösti

Add streaky bacon, cut in small strips or cubes (you will find packs of diced bacon in the chiller cabinet of many continental supermarkets).

Basilean Rösti

Use half potatoes and half sliced onions.

Valaisian Rösti

Once the rösti has cooked; place sliced tomatoes and some Raclette cheese (or any easily melted strongly flavored cheese) over the top. When the cheese has melted, serve with the crust on the bottom instead of flipping it over.

Mediterranean Rösti

Use half olive oil and half butter, add chopped fresh rosemary to the potatoes and grind a little black pepper over them.

CHECK ALL ingredient labels EVERY TIME YOU BUY

Lyonnaise potatoes
4 Servings
500g (1 lb) potatoes, sliced thinly
250g (½ lb) onions, peeled and sliced very thinly
275ml (½ UK pint, 1¼ US cups) stock
60g (2 oz) grated cheese

Preheat oven to 180°C (350°F, gas mark 4).

Butter a shallow ovenproof dish and make alternate layers of potatoes and onions until full, finishing with potatoes.

Pour over the stock and top with grated cheese.

Cover and cook for 1¼ hours. Remove cover and cook for a further 15 minutes until golden brown.

Serve hot. Goes well with partridge, goose or turkey.

Duchesse potatoes
6 Servings
700g (1½ lb) potatoes
45g (1½ oz) butter
2 egg yolks
salt and black pepper
beaten egg for baking

If preparing for immediate use, pre-heat oven to 190°C (375°F, gas mark 5).

Peel, cook and mash potatoes. Stir in butter and egg yolks, season with salt and pepper.

Put into a piping bag with a large rose nozzle and pipe whirls onto a greased baking tray. Alternatively, scoop onto tray and shape with spoon.

(To freeze, place tray in freezer before baking and open freeze before removing from tray and packing away.)

Brush with beaten egg and bake for 10 minutes until golden brown.

Serve hot.

CHECK ALL ingredient labels EVERY TIME YOU BUY

To serve from the freezer, place the potatoes on a baking tray and thaw for 1-2 hours. Brush with beaten egg and bake in the oven at 190°C (375°F, gas mark 5) for about 10 minutes until golden brown. Serve hot.

Alu ko kufte (Nepali potato kebabs)
6 Servings

12 large potatoes
4 spring (green) onions
1 cup chopped coriander
1 cup peeled mashed tomatoes
2 cups cooked cauliflower
juice of 1 lime
oil
salt

Chop spring (green) onions and cauliflower. Boil potatoes in salted water and mash until smooth.

In a separate bowl, mix remaining ingredients except oil.

Divide mashed potato into small balls, stuff with mixture and flatten.

Heat oil and fry until brown. Serve hot.

Cox's Orange cauliflower
6 Servings

500g (1 lb) cauliflower florets
90g (3 oz) butter
2 large Cox's apples, peeled, cored and sliced

Cook cauliflower. Drain and keep hot.

Melt butter in a saucepan, add apple and fry gently for about 10 minutes until golden. Add cauliflower and cook, turning frequently, until golden.

Serve hot. Excellent with pork, pigeon or goose.

CHECK ALL ingredient labels EVERY TIME YOU BUY

Ratatouille

6 Servings

6 tblsp olive oil
2 large onions, peeled and sliced
350g (12 oz) tomatoes, peeled and sliced
2 large aubergines (eggplants), sliced
2 medium green peppers, de-seeded and sliced
2 large courgettes (zucchini), sliced
2 cloves garlic, crushed
2 level tsp salt
black pepper

Heat oil gently in a large frying pan. Fry onion for 5-7 minutes until translucent.

Add remaining ingredients, cover and cook for 1 hour over a very low heat, stirring from time to time.

Serve hot or cold.

DESSERTS AND PUDDINGS

Grapefruit sorbet
8 Servings
180g (6 oz) caster sugar
2 tblsp water
850ml (1½ UK pints, 3⅞ US cups) grapefruit juice
2 egg whites
2-3 drops of red coloring
mint sprig to garnish

Combine sugar and water in a saucepan. Heat gently to dissolve sugar. Cool, add grapefruit juice and stir to mix.

Pour into a shallow plastic box with a fitting lid. Put into freezer and leave for about 2-4 hours until just freezing.

Stiffly whip egg whites.

Turn sorbet into a bowl and mash with a fork until smooth. Fold in egg whites and add coloring to make it a pale pink. Put back into the container and store in the freezer until required. Use within 3 months.

Variation: Lemon sorbet
8 Servings
180g (6 oz) caster sugar
550ml (1 UK pint, 2½ US cups) water
2 egg whites
275ml (½ UK pint, 1¼ US cups) pure lemon juice
grated rind of 1 lemon

Omit the coloring.

Make as for grapefruit sorbet, using 2 tblsp of the measured amount of water to dissolve the sugar. Add the lemon rind with the juice and remaining water.

CHECK ALL ingredient labels EVERY TIME YOU BUY

Apple lemon mousse

6 Servings

1 packet lemon jelly (jello)
275ml (½ UK pint, 1¼ US cups) unsweetened apple
    purée
2 eggs, separated
1 lemon

Dissolve the jelly and make up to 250ml (½ pint) with boiling water.

Mix apple purée and egg yolks with the grated rind of half a lemon. Stir in the jelly and put in a cold place to cool.

When the jelly mixture is almost set, stiffly whisk egg whites.

Whisk the mixture until thick and pale, then fold in egg whites. Pour into a serving dish.

Decorate with lemon slices from the remaining half of the lemon and serve chilled.

Coffee ginger surprise

6 Servings

4 egg whites
125g (4 oz) granulated sugar
125g (4 oz) caster sugar
550ml (1 UK pint, 2½ US cups) double (heavy) cream
275ml (½ UK pint, 1¼ US cups) coffee ice cream
2 tblsp stem ginger, chopped
sliced stem ginger to decorate

Preheat oven to lowest setting.

Beat egg whites stiffly. Gradually add granulated sugar, beat again. Fold in caster sugar.

Divide and form into 3 rounds, 15cm (6") in diameter on a non-stick baking tray. Bake for 2 hours until the meringue is dry. Cool.

Whip cream until softly stiff. Add chopped ginger to half the cream and set the remainder to one side.

CHECK ALL ingredient labels EVERY TIME YOU BUY

Cover one round with ice cream, place on top of second round. Spread with ginger cream, place third round on top.

Spread top and sides with reserved cream. Decorate with stem ginger and serve immediately.

Grapefruit freeze

4 Servings

2 grapefruit
375g (13 oz, 2½ US cups) low fat gluten free yogurt
3 tsp clear honey
1 sprig fresh mint

Cut grapefruit in half, scoop out flesh and cut into pieces, discarding the segment skins and pips.

Mix yogurt and honey well, then stir in grapefruit and pile the mixture back into the empty grapefruit halves.

Open freeze. Can be stored by wrapping in the usual way for use within 2 months.

To serve, thaw for 30 minutes in a refrigerator. Serve still partially frozen, garnished with fresh mint leaves.

Grape brûlée

2 Servings

500g (1 lb) grapes
2 tblsp brandy
550ml (1 UK pint, 2½ US cups) double (heavy) cream
1 tblsp soft brown sugar

Seedless grapes are the best, but if yours aren't, remove seeds with a sharp pointed knife.

Divide the grapes between two crème caramel dishes. Sprinkle with the brandy.

Whip the cream until it is stiff and cover the grapes with it.

Sprinkle with the sugar and freeze for 1 hour.

Remove from the freezer and place under a hot grill until the sugar bubbles. Serve immediately.

CHECK ALL ingredient labels EVERY TIME YOU BUY

Gooseberry ice cream

8 Servings

4 eggs, separated
125g (4 oz) caster sugar
275ml (½ UK pint, 1¼ US cups) double (heavy) cream
125g (4 oz) gooseberries
1 level tblsp sugar

Cook gooseberries with 1 tblsp sugar until soft. Cool. Purée in a blender.

Beat yolks in a small bowl until thoroughly blended. Whisk cream to the soft peak stage.

In a large mixing bowl, whisk egg whites until stiff. Beat in sugar gradually, 1 tsp at a time.

Pour in egg yolks and fold in gently. Fold in the cream.

Add flavoring and mix thoroughly.

Pour into a 2½ pint shallow container with a fitting lid.

Freeze.

After 2 hours, when it is partly frozen, break up with a fork and mix well. Return to freezer.

Iced zabaglione

4 Servings

4 egg yolks
125g (4 oz) caster sugar
190ml (6 fl oz, ¾ US cup) Marsala
angelica and glacé cherries to decorate (optional)

Beat the egg yolks to a pale cream and mix in the sugar and Marsala.

Cook in a double saucepan or a bowl over a pan of boiling water, stirring continuously, until the custard coats the back of the spoon.

Pour into individual ramekin dishes and cool.

Freeze until firm. Decorate with angelica and cherries if

CHECK ALL ingredient labels EVERY TIME YOU BUY

desired.

Serve with crisp wafer or boudoir biscuits.

Raspberry sorbet

6 Servings

180g (6 oz) caster sugar
550ml (1 UK pint, 2½ US cups) water
2 egg whites
500g (1 lb) raspberries

Combine sugar and water in a saucepan. Heat gently to dissolve sugar. Cool. Liquidize raspberries and add to sugar water, mix well. Stiffly whip egg whites.

Pour into a shallow plastic box with a fitting lid. Put into freezer and leave for about 2-4 hours until just freezing.

Turn sorbet into a bowl and mash with a fork until smooth. Fold in egg whites. Put back into the container and store in the freezer until required. Use within 3 months.

Coffee mousse

6 Servings

3 large eggs
60g (2 oz) soft brown sugar
15g (½ oz) gelatine
2 level tblsp instant coffee
3 tblsp boiling water
275ml (½ UK pint, 1¼ US cups) double (heavy) cream

Separate eggs and whisk yolks and sugar in a basin over hot water until thickened.

Soak gelatine. Blend coffee powder and water. Stir into gelatine until dissolved. Stir into egg yolk mixture.

Whip cream until stiff and fold into mixture.

Whip egg whites until stiff and fold in.

Transfer to serving dish, refrigerate until set.

Serve decorated with whipped cream and grated chocolate.

CHECK ALL ingredient labels EVERY TIME YOU BUY

Hazelnut and apple mousse
4-6 Servings

2 tblsp lemon juice
500g (1 lb) eating apples
60g (2 oz) chopped hazelnuts
15g (½ oz) gelatine
4 egg whites
green coloring
60g (2 oz) sugar
4 tblsp double (heavy) cream

Put the lemon juice into a saucepan. Peel, core and grate the apples and mix together.

Cook gently until very soft. Remove from the heat and stir in half the nuts.

Dissolve the gelatine in 1 tblsp of water in a basin over a pan of simmering water. Stir into apple mixture.

Whisk egg whites until stiff, gradually adding coloring until it turns pale green. Whisk in sugar.

Fold egg mixture into apple and put into a serving dish. Decorate with whipped cream and the remaining nuts.

Serve chilled.

Loganberry whip
4 Servings

250g (8 oz) loganberries
150ml (¼ UK pint, ⅝ US cup) water
2 level tblsp granulated sugar
1 raspberry jelly (jello) mix
190ml (6 fl oz, ¾ US cup) evaporated milk
1 tsp lemon juice

Cook fruit gently until soft. Add sugar and stir.

Strain the juice and put into a saucepan. Bring back to the boil and add the jelly mix in cubes, stirring until dissolved.

CHECK ALL ingredient labels EVERY TIME YOU BUY

Pour into a measure and make up to 250ml (½ pint) with cold water if necessary. Cool.

Whisk the evaporated milk and lemon juice together until thickening and forming peaks.

Purée loganberries in a blender and fold into the mixture, along with the cooled jelly mix. Mix well and pour into a basin.

Put in the refrigerator to set.

Serve with whipped cream.

Winter fruit salad
6 Servings

550ml (1 UK pint, 2½ US cups) water
2 tblsp clear honey
a pinch of cinnamon
2 cloves
juice of half a lemon
175g (6 oz) dried apricots
125g (4 oz) dried prunes
125g (4 oz) dried figs
60g (2 oz) raisins
30g (1 oz) walnut pieces, coarsely chopped

Put apricots, prunes and figs in a large bowl, cover with plenty of boiling water, to about 10cm (4") above the level of the fruit. Leave to soak overnight.

Drain fruit.

Put the measured water, honey, cinnamon and cloves in a pan and bring to the boil. Add lemon juice and soaked fruit.

Cover and simmer gently for 10 minutes. Add raisins and simmer for 2-3 minutes. Remove cloves and discard.

Spoon into individual dishes and sprinkle with walnuts. Serve hot or cold, with cream if liked.

CHECK ALL ingredient labels EVERY TIME YOU BUY

RECIPES KIDS LOVE

Ali Baba pears
4 Servings

8 peeled cored pear halves
550ml (1 UK pint, 2½ US cups) orange juice
pinch cinnamon powder

Preheat oven to 140°C (gas mark 1, 275°F).

Lay pear halves in an ovenproof dish, mix orange juice, water and cinnamon powder together and pour over. Bake for 2 hours.

Blueberry cheesecake
Makes 22cm cheesecake

500g (1 lb) cream cheese
125g (4 oz) sugar
2 drops vanilla essence
2 eggs
1 can gluten free blueberry pie filling
a quarter of a pack of rice bran crackers
60g (2 oz) butter

Preheat oven to 180°C (350°F, gas mark 4).

Crush the crackers. Melt the butter and mix into the crackers. Use the mixture to line the base of a 22cm loose bottom cake tin.

Mix together cream cheese, sugar and vanilla until smooth. Beat the eggs lightly. Add to cream cheese mixture and mix well. Pour the mixture over the cracker mixture.

Spoon one third of the can of pie filling onto mixture and gently swirl.

Bake for 40 minutes or until the centre is set. Cool to room temperature and then refrigerate. Top with remaining pie filling if desired.

CHECK ALL ingredient labels EVERY TIME YOU BUY

Apple snow

4 Servings

500g (1 lb) cooking apples, peeled and chopped
2 level tblsp caster sugar
1 level tsp grated lemon rind
2 eggs, separated
150ml (¼ UK pint, $\frac{5}{8}$ US cup) double (heavy) cream

Cook apple, sugar and lemon rind together with a very small amount of water if needed, to make a purée.

Remove from the heat and stir the egg yolks in quickly. The mixture should thicken.

Allow to cool and pour into a bowl.

Beat the egg whites until stiff and in another bowl whip the cream. Fold the egg white gently into the mixture, followed by the cream.

Refrigerate for at least 30 minutes before serving.

Blackberry ice cream

8 Servings

600g (1¼ lb) blackberries
1 tsp lemon juice
4 eggs
125g (4 oz) caster sugar
4 drops vanilla essence
550ml (1 UK pint, 2½ US cups) double (heavy) cream

Place blackberries and lemon juice in a blender and liquidize.

Combine eggs, sugar and vanilla in a bowl. Beat until fluffy. Fold in the puréed fruit.

Lightly whip the cream and fold into the mixture.

Turn into a rigid container and seal. Rapid freeze for 10 hours. Remove 2 hours before serving. Serve with Fresh Fruit Salad or Exotic Fruit Salad.

CHECK ALL ingredient labels EVERY TIME YOU BUY

Coffee ice cream

8 Servings

4 eggs, separated
125g (4 oz) caster sugar
275ml (½ UK pint, 1¼ US cups) double (heavy) cream
2 tsp instant coffee
1 tblsp boiling water

Dissolve the coffee in the boiling water and leave to cool.

Beat yolks in a small bowl until thoroughly blended.

Whisk cream to the soft peak stage.

In a large mixing bowl, whisk egg whites until stiff. Beat in sugar gradually, 1 tsp at a time.

Pour in egg yolks and fold in gently. Fold in the cream.

Add flavoring and mix thoroughly.

Pour into a 1½ litre (2½ pint) shallow container with a fitting lid.

Freeze.

After 2 hours, when it is partly frozen, break up with a fork and mix well. Return to freezer.

Chocolate orange mousse

8 Servings

250g (8 oz) plain chocolate
3 tsp gelatine
4 tblsp hot water
550ml (1 UK pint, 2½ US cups) double (heavy) cream
6 eggs, separated
half an orange, grated rind and juice
whipped cream to decorate

Melt chocolate.

Dissolve gelatine in the hot water.

Beat cream until thick, add yolks and beat in. Fold in melted chocolate. Stir in gelatine, orange rind and juice.

CHECK ALL ingredient labels EVERY TIME YOU BUY

Leave aside until almost set.

Beat egg whites until stiff. Fold into mixture.

Transfer to serving dishes and leave to set for 1 hour.

Decorate with whipped cream. Serve chilled.

Chocolate pots
Makes 6

3 eggs, separated
180g (6 oz) dark chocolate (about 80% cocoa)
275ml (½ UK pint, 1¼ US cups) whipping cream

Whisk egg whites until stiff.

Melt chocolate in microwave or in a bowl over a pan of hot water. Stir in 2 tblsp cream.

Beat in the egg yolks and fold in the whites.

Divide mixture between 6 individual ramekins. Chill.

Top with whipped cream and serve.

Fresh fruit salad
8 Servings

450g (12 oz) melon or grapes, seeds removed
250g (8 oz) fresh pineapple
250g (8 oz) apricots or kiwi fruit
125g (4 oz) mandarin segments or strawberries
200ml (8 fl oz, 1 US cup) orange, apple or grape juice

Cut all the fruit into similar sized pieces (large grapes can be cut in half, smaller ones left whole). Cover with the fruit juice and leave in the refrigerator overnight to allow the flavors to blend.

Serve with real or fake cream.

CHECK ALL ingredient labels EVERY TIME YOU BUY

Exotic fruit salad
8-10 Servings

570ml (1 UK pint, 2½ US cups) water
180g (6 oz) sugar
2 tblsp lemon juice
250g (½ lb) blackberries
250g (½ lb) raspberries
250g (½ lb) strawberries
125g (¼ lb) grapes, deseeded
4 fresh figs, sliced
250g (½ lb) lychees, peeled
60ml (2 fl oz, ¼ US cup) orange liqueur

Combine water and sugar in a heavy pan and bring slowly to the boil, making sure sugar dissolves. Boil steadily until reduced by half. Add lemon juice and orange liqueur. Cool.

Prepare fruit and combine in a large bowl. Pour over the syrup.

Chill and serve with Blackberry Ice Cream.

Pineapple sorbet
6 Servings

180g (6 oz) caster sugar
570ml (1 UK pint, 2½ US cups) water
2 egg whites
1 medium sized pineapple

Cut the top off the pineapple and scoop out the flesh. Liquidize until smooth.

Combine sugar and water in a saucepan. Heat gently to dissolve sugar. Cool. Add pineapple purée to sugarwater, mix well.

Pour into a shallow plastic box with a fitting lid. Put into freezer and leave for about 2-4 hours until just freezing.

Stiffly whip egg whites.

Turn sorbet into a bowl and mash with a fork until

CHECK ALL ingredient labels EVERY TIME YOU BUY

smooth. Fold in egg whites. Put back into the container and store in the freezer until required. Use within 3 months. If using the same day, pile the sorbet into the pineapple and serve into individual dishes at table.

Gooseberry fool
6 Servings

1 kg (2 lb) gooseberries
375g (12 oz) caster sugar
1 egg white
275ml (½ UK pint, 1¼ US cups) double (heavy) cream

Cook gooseberries and sugar over a low heat until soft.

Remove from heat and blend until smooth. Cool.

Whip egg whites until stiff. Fold into fruit.

Whip cream until stiff and fold most of it into the fruit mixture, reserving a small quantity for decoration.

Spoon into dishes and top with cream.

Orange sorbet
8 Servings

180g (6 oz) caster sugar
2 tblsp water
850ml (1½ UK pints, 3¾ UK cups) orange juice
2 egg whites
mint sprig to garnish

Combine sugar and water in a saucepan. Heat gently to dissolve sugar. Cool, add orange juice and stir to mix.

Pour into a shallow plastic box with a fitting lid. Put into freezer and leave for about 2-4 hours until just freezing.

Stiffly whip egg whites.

Turn sorbet into a bowl and mash with a fork until smooth. Fold in egg whites. Put back into the container and store in the freezer until required. Use within 3 months.

CHECK ALL ingredient labels EVERY TIME YOU BUY

Sweet pancakes

3 Servings (3 pancakes each)

275ml (½ UK pint, 1¼ US cups) milk
1-2 eggs
a small pinch of salt
115g (3½ oz) rice flour
Oil to fry

Suggested fillings:
Traditional: Sugar and lemon
Maple syrup
Jam
Apple purée

Put the milk and eggs with the salt into a large jug and beat to break up the eggs. Sprinkle on the flour and mix in with a whisk, one tablespoonful at a time. Leave to stand for about 10 minutes, then stir again with the whisk so that the flour is evenly distributed (and not in a sticky mass at the bottom).

Using a small frying pan about the size of the pancakes you want (about 20cm diameter), heat a very small amount of oil to coat the base completely. Pour off excess oil into a saucer.

Pour a small quantity of the batter into the pan, about half as much as it seems you need. Tip the pan to coat the base evenly. Cook for a minute or so until little holes appear all over and the edges turn brown and start to curl up.

Using a palette knife, loosen the edges of the pancake and flip it over to cook the other side. Turn out onto a plate and cover with a clean dry cloth to keep warm.

Add a little more oil and tip out as before (you can use the oil from the saucer if there is enough). Pour in a similar amount of batter and repeat the process as described, stacking the pancakes on top of each other on the plate and covering with the cloth.

When all the pancakes are cooked, put one at a time

CHECK ALL ingredient labels EVERY TIME YOU BUY

onto a plate, add the filling at one end or spread thinly on one side and roll up, then transfer to plate for serving.

Strawberry mousse

6 Servings

750g (1½ lb) strawberries
3 large eggs, separated
150g (5 oz) caster sugar
15g (½ oz) powdered gelatine
3 tblsp cold water
275ml (½ UK pint, 1¼ US cups) double (heavy) cream
2-3 drops red coloring

Pick over strawberries, removing stalks. Select 12 attractive ones and set aside. Blend the remainder to a purée.

Whip half of the cream lightly.

Prepare a 500ml (1¼ pint) soufflé dish: fix a double piece of greaseproof paper, about 5cm (2") deeper than the dish, firmly around the outside, to form a collar and tie with string.

Whisk the egg yolks and sugar in a basin over a pan of hot water until they are beginning to thicken.

Mix gelatine with water, and dissolve in a bowl over a pan of simmering water.

Stir gelatine and strawberry purée into egg and sugar mixture. Remove from heat and leave to cool until it begins to thicken, stirring occasionally.

Fold in the whipped cream, followed by the stiffly whisked egg whites. Add coloring and stir well to mix.

Pour into the soufflé dish and leave to set in the refrigerator for 2-3 hours.

Remove collar carefully using a knife. Whisk remaining cream and pipe on top. Decorate with reserved strawberries.

CHECK ALL ingredient labels EVERY TIME YOU BUY

Fruit kebabs
Makes 6 (2-3 Servings)

3 bananas
2 apples
2 kiwi fruit
1 425g (14 oz) can pineapple chunks, drained
1 punnet strawberries
juice of 1 lemon

You will need 6 skewers. If using wooden or bamboo ones, soak them in cold water for 15 minutes.

Peel bananas, apples and kiwi fruit and cut into pieces, skewer together along with the pineapple and strawberries. Sprinkle all surfaces with lemon juice to prevent discoloration.

Serve with gluten free Melba sauce or chocolate sauce and/or whipped cream.

Pear and almond flan
8 Servings

Pastry
180g (6 oz) potato flour
60g (2 oz) rice flour
120g (4 oz) softened butter
90g (3 oz) caster sugar
1 egg

Filling
4 fresh pears
160ml (5 fl oz) water for poaching
60g (2 oz) Demerara (Turbinado) sugar
1½ tblsp lemon juice
45g (1½ oz) icing sugar
45g (1½ oz) caster sugar
90g (3 oz) ground almonds
60g (2 oz) soft butter or margarine
1 egg

CHECK ALL ingredient labels EVERY TIME YOU BUY

Glaze
3 tblsp warmed apricot jam, sieved

Put all the pastry ingredients into a bowl and work together until a dough is formed (use an electric mixer or wooden spoon). Dust with rice flour, flatten into a block about 25mm (1") thick and wrap in foil. Chill overnight in fridge.

Preheat oven to 180°C (350°F, gas mark 4).

In a large pan dissolve the sugar in the water and lemon juice. Peel and core pears and cut in half. Add them in single layers and baste. Cover and simmer until tender - about 15 minutes. Lift out and drain on paper towels. (The poaching liquid can be saved and used for poaching other fruit or for a fruit salad).

Roll out the pastry and use to line a 26cm (10") flan tin. Prick well all over. Don't worry if it breaks, just patch it up - it will not be noticed when cooked. Put in freezer.

Mix together remaining filling ingredients to make frangipane.

Remove pastry from freezer. Put frangipane mixture on base. Cut nicks round the pears at 1cm (½") intervals, making sure not to cut through, and place on top of the frangipane mixture. Press gently on each pear - it should spread like a fan - then paint with heated jam.

Bake for 30-35 minutes until pastry is golden brown. Serve at room temperature.

Will keep for 2 days in the fridge.

CHECK ALL ingredient labels EVERY TIME YOU BUY

Vanilla ice cream
8 Servings

4 eggs, separated
125g (4 oz) caster sugar
275ml (½ UK pint, 1¼ US cups) double (heavy) cream
2-3 drops vanilla essence

Beat yolks in a small bowl until thoroughly blended.

Whisk cream to the soft peak stage.

In a large mixing bowl, whisk egg whites until stiff. Beat in sugar gradually, 1 tsp at a time.

Pour in egg yolks and fold in gently. Fold in the cream.

Add flavoring and mix thoroughly.

Pour into a 2½ pint shallow container with a fitting lid.

Freeze.

After 2 hours, when it is partly frozen, break up with a fork and mix well. Return to freezer.

Banana split
2 Servings

2 ripe bananas
4 scoops vanilla ice cream
Gluten free chocolate sauce or Melba sauce
Whipped cream (optional)
A few chopped hazelnuts (optional)

Prepare immediately before serving, or the bananas will go brown and become unappetising.

Peel the bananas and cut in half lengthwise. Arrange each in a suitable dish or on a large plate. Put 2 scoops of ice cream between the bananas, cover with whipped cream. if used. Drizzle with sauce, sprinkle with nuts if liked and serve.

CHECK ALL ingredient labels EVERY TIME YOU BUY

Sultana Cheesecake
Makes a 22cm cheesecake

Base:
100-125g (3-4 oz) gluten free biscuits
60g (2 oz) butter
Filling:
60g (2 oz) sultanas
150g (5 oz) butter or olive margarine
150g (5 oz) cream cheese.
150g (5 oz) caster sugar
150g (5 oz) ground almonds
5 eggs, separated
30g (1 oz) maize flour
juice and finely grated rind of 1 lemon

If possible, soak sultanas overnight in enough hot water to cover. Drain. Preheat oven to 200°C (400°F, gas mark 6).

Break biscuits into crumbs in a blender or wrap in a clean cloth and bash repeatedly with a rolling pin.

Melt butter, stir in the biscuit crumbs. Spread evenly over the bottom of a loose bottomed 22cm (9") cake tin.

Beat butter and sugar for the filling. Beat in the cream cheese followed by the egg yolks. Fold in the maize flour, lemon juice and rind, and ground almonds.

Beat the egg whites until stiff and fold into mixture.

Cover the base with the drained sultanas, then pour the filling over the top and spread evenly.

Bake for 15 minutes. Turn the heat down to 180°C (350°F, gas mark 4) and bake for a further 25-30 minutes.

Cool and serve. Can be stored in the freezer for 3-4 months.

CHECK ALL ingredient labels EVERY TIME YOU BUY

DESSERTS AND PUDDINGS: ACCOMPANIMENTS

Brandy butter
8 Servings

125g (4 oz) caster sugar
60ml (2 fl oz) brandy
125g (4 oz) butter, softened

Put sugar in bowl, add brandy and stir until sugar is completely dissolved.

Put the butter into the bowl with the brandy and sugar, and mix thoroughly.

Transfer to a serving dish. Chill. Traditionally served with Christmas pudding.

Butterscotch rum sauce
6-8 Servings

3 tblsp golden syrup
3 level tblsp brown sugar
45g (1½ oz) butter
600ml (1 pint) milk
2 level tblsp cornflour (cornstarch) or arrowroot
1 tblsp lemon juice
2 tblsp rum

Heat syrup, sugar and butter together in a small thick saucepan until it starts caramelising.

Blend the milk and cornflour or arrowroot to a smooth cream. Add to the saucepan, stirring continuously and stir until thickened.

Stir in lemon juice and rum. Serve hot.

CHECK ALL ingredient labels EVERY TIME YOU BUY

Tangy summer sauce
6-8 Servings

60g (2 oz) butter
60g (2 oz) caster sugar
2 eggs, beaten
juice of 1 orange
150ml (¼ UK pint, $\frac{5}{8}$ US cup) pineapple juice
1 level tsp cornflour (cornstarch) or arrowroot

Melt the butter. Add sugar, beaten eggs, and fruit juices, made up to 300ml with cold water.

Cook together until hot, stirring now and then.

Blend cornflour or arrowroot with a little water and add, stirring continuously until thickened. Serve hot with South Seas Christmas pudding.

CHECK ALL ingredient labels EVERY TIME YOU BUY

RECIPES KIDS LOVE

Blueberry sauce
Makes about 300ml

65g (2½ oz) sugar
1 tblsp cornflour (cornstarch)
95ml (3½ fl oz, ⅜ US cup) water
2 tblsp lemon juice
225g (8 oz) fresh or frozen blueberries

Put all the ingredients in a pan and cook over medium heat, stirring continuously, until thickened.

Can be stored in a covered container in the refrigerator for 2-3 days.

This goes extremely well with pancakes or ice cream.

California sauce
6-8 Servings

400ml (13½ oz) can prunes, stoned and chopped
1 orange, rind and juice
1 lemon, rind and juice
1 level tblsp cornflour (cornstarch) or arrowroot
2 tblsp water

Combine prunes and juice in a pan with fruit rinds and juices. Bring to the boil.

Blend cornflour or arrowroot with water, and stir into the hot mixture until evenly mixed and thickened. Serve hot.

Melba sauce
8 Servings

500g (1 lb) raspberries
60g (2 oz) sugar
1 level tblsp cornflour (cornstarch) or arrowroot

This recipe was especially created by the Head Chef at the Ritz Hotel, London for the then very famous actress, Nelly Melba.

CHECK ALL ingredient labels EVERY TIME YOU BUY

Wash and hull raspberries. Cook gently with the sugar for about 10 minutes. Blend or sieve to a purée.

Mix cornflour or arrowroot with a little water to make a smooth cream. Stir into sauce. Reheat, stirring continuously, until the mixture thickens and becomes translucent.

Serve over poached peaches or with vanilla ice cream.

Chocolate sauce for ice cream
8 Servings

60g (2 oz) dark chocolate
375ml (12 fl oz, 1½ US cups) water
225g (7 oz) caster sugar
1 tblsp cornflour (cornstarch) or arrowroot
a pinch of salt

Break chocolate into pieces. Put in a small saucepan with the water and stir over a low heat until smooth.

Add sugar, cornflour and salt. Cook until sugar is dissolved and sauce thickened.

Bring to the boil and cook for 3 minutes.

Serve hot with ice cream.

CHECK ALL ingredient labels EVERY TIME YOU BUY

CAKES, BAKES AND SWEETIES

Almond cookies (Macaroons)
Makes 16

1 egg white
75g (3 oz) ground almonds
100g (3½ oz) caster sugar
¼ tsp almond essence
16 whole blanched almonds
rice paper

Preheat oven to 180°C (350°F, gas mark 4). Line a couple of large baking sheets with rice paper.

Whisk the egg whites until very stiff. Fold in the ground almonds and almond essence.

Spoon small mounds (about 2.5cm/1" in size) spaced well apart to allow for spreading onto the rice paper. Top each with an almond.

Bake for 20-25 minutes until a pale gold or dark cream color.

Lift the whole sheet onto a rack to cool.

When cold, tear apart, remove excess paper and discard. Pack cookies in an airtight container or serve.

Mocha cake
Makes a 23cm cake

4 eggs, separated
180g (6 oz) caster sugar
45g (1½ oz) potato flour
15g (½ oz) cocoa
1 tblsp hot coffee

Filling
150ml (¼ UK pint, $\frac{5}{8}$ US cup) double (heavy) cream
1 tblsp cold strong coffee
2 tsp caster sugar

Preheat oven to 180°C (350°F, gas mark 4).

CHECK ALL ingredient labels EVERY TIME YOU BUY

Whisk egg yolks until creamy, then add caster sugar, and continue whisking until the mixture forms a thick ribbon as it falls from the beater.

Sieve potato flour and cocoa together and add to yolk mixture. Add hot coffee. Fold in egg whites.

Spoon into two 23cm (9") loose bottomed cake tin, which have been greased, then dusted with rice flour.

Bake for 30 minutes, then reduce heat to 170°C (325°F, gas mark 3) and cook for 20 minutes. Turn oven to its lowest setting for a further 10 minutes, then turn the heat off altogether and leave the cake in the oven for a final 10 minutes before removing.

Turn out and cool on a wire tray.

Whisk cream until it holds its shape, add coffee and sugar. Fill cake.

Dust with icing sugar and serve.

Banana cake
Makes 1 loaf cake

1 ripe banana.
60g (2 oz) softened butter
1 large egg
120g (4 oz) Demerara (Turbinado) sugar
½ tsp vanilla extract
30g (1 oz) rice flour
90g (3 oz) potato flour
30g (1 oz) ground almonds
¼ tsp bicarbonate of soda
1 tsp gluten free baking powder

Preheat oven to 180°C (350°F, gas mark 4).

Liquidize the first five ingredients together.

Add to remaining ingredients and mix well.

Turn into a greased and lined loaf tin and bake for 30-35 minutes.

Turn out and cool on a wire tray. Can be stored in the freezer for up to 3 months.

CHECK ALL ingredient labels EVERY TIME YOU BUY

Mock oatmeal cookies
100-110 cookies

480g (17 oz) butter, room temperature
450g (1 lb) white sugar
225g (8 oz) brown sugar
2 eggs
500g (18 oz) rice flour
70g (2½ oz) potato flour
20g (1 oz, ¼ US cup) gram flour (besan/chickpea
    flour/garbanzo flour)
1 tsp salt
2 tsp bicarbonate of soda
2 tsp gluten free baking powder
2 cups flaked almonds

Preheat oven to 190°C (375°F, gas mark 5).

Cream together the butter, sugar and eggs. Sift dry ingredients and mix in. Stir in the flaked almonds.

Drop rounded tablespoonfuls onto greased or lined baking sheets.

Bake for 7-10 minutes, until light brown.

Transfer to a rack and allow to cool.

Store in an airtight container. Can be frozen.

CHECK ALL ingredient labels EVERY TIME YOU BUY

RECIPES KIDS LOVE

Almond berries

350g (12 oz) ground almonds
115g (4 oz) icing sugar
Rosewater
55g (2 oz) pistachio nuts, cut into slivers

Make a stiff paste with the almonds, sugar and rosewater. Divide into small portions and roll into elongated berry shapes. Add a pistachio stalk.

Store in an airtight container to prevent them drying out.

Apricot no-bake cookies
Makes 40

60g (2 oz) icing sugar, sieved
60g (2 oz) caster sugar
60g (2 oz) ground almonds
90g (3 oz) ground rice
1 egg, beaten
1 tsp lemon juice
4 drops almond essence
1 tblsp apricot jam
60g (2 oz) dried apricots, finely chopped
30g (1 oz) hazelnuts, finely chopped

Mix together sugars, almonds and ground rice. Add egg, lemon juice and essence. Blend to a stiff paste. Divide into two.

Roll out each half to 8"x5" on a sugared board. Brush with warmed jam and sprinkle with apricots. Roll up like a Swiss roll. Coat with hazelnuts.

Wrap in foil and chill for half an hour. Cut into slices to serve.

CHECK ALL ingredient labels EVERY TIME YOU BUY

Fuzzy fruit boulders

Makes 20

300g (½ lb) dried apricots
250g (6 oz) raisins
250g (6 oz) sultanas
1 tblsp honey
100g (3 oz) shredded coconut

Chop all the fruit into small pieces or blend for a short time, but only until they are roughly cut into similar sized pieces.

Put into a bowl, add honey and half the coconut. Mix well.

Shape into about 20 balls, roll in remaining coconut.

Store in a covered container in the refrigerator.

Angel Food cake

16 servings

15 egg whites, at room temperature
75g (2½ oz) potato flour
75g (2½ oz) cornflour (cornstarch)
400g (14 oz) sugar
½ tsp salt
½ tsp cream of tartar
1 tsp vanilla extract
1 tsp almond extract

Bring egg whites to room temperature. Preheat oven to 180°C (350°F, gas mark 4).

Sift together the potato flour, cornflour, and 175g (6 oz) sugar. Set aside.

Sift remaining sugar separately.

In a large bowl combine the egg whites, salt, cream of tartar, vanilla and almond extracts.

Beat on high speed until stiff and standing in peaks. This takes 1½ to 2 minutes. Be careful not to overdo it.

CHECK ALL ingredient labels EVERY TIME YOU BUY

Run the mixer on medium speed whilst quickly sprinkling in the remaining sugar - about 1 minute.

Turn mixer to lowest speed and sprinkle in the sifted flour mixture - 1½ minutes.

Pour cake mixture into the ungreased 10 inch tube pan.

Bake for 35 minutes. It is better to bake for a little too long rather than underbake.

Remove from oven and turn upside down on the worktop to cool.

Chilled lemon cheesecake
8 servings

Base:
175g (6 oz) gluten free biscuits
50g (2 oz) butter
½-1 tsp cinnamon

Filling:
250g (9 oz) low fat cream cheese
175ml (6 fl oz) sweetened condensed milk
grated rind and juice of 2 lemons
150ml (5 fl oz) cream, stiffly whipped

Either use a blender to crush the biscuits, or wrap them inside a clean towel and use a rolling pin.

Melt the butter and add the crushed biscuit and the cinnamon. Mix well and use to line the base of a 23cm (9½") loose bottomed cake tin. Put in the refrigerator to become firm.

Mix the cream cheese, lemon rind and juice and condensed milk thoroughly. Fold in the stiffly whipped cream.

Pour the mixture on the chilled biscuit base. It will be quite liquid at this stage.

Chill for at least an hour before serving, preferably overnight.

CHECK ALL ingredient labels EVERY TIME YOU BUY

Popcorn with candy coating
A big bowlful

1 tblsp oil
60g (2 oz) popping corn
60g (2 oz) butter
4 tblsp golden syrup

Put oil into a large pan with a tight fitting lid and heat until a haze appears. Put the corn into the lid of the pan, tip into the oil and clamp the lid on immediately.

Cook over a high heat, holding the lid on and shaking continuously until the popping noise has stopped. Turn off the heat, pull pan to one side and allow to cool for about 30 seconds before removing lid. Pour the corn into a bowl.

In the pan you used to cook the corn, heat the butter and syrup together until the butter melts and the mixture is bubbling well.

Return the corn to the pan and stir until it is well coated, then transfer to a lightly greased tray to cool.

When cold, store in an airtight container.

Chocolate fudge
Makes 1.5 kg

250g (½ lb) plain chocolate
250g (½ lb) butter
1 kg (2 lb) granulated sugar
570ml (1 UK pint, 2½ US cups) can evaporated milk
275ml (½ UK pint, 1¼ US cups) water

Melt chocolate.

Heat butter, sugar, milk and water in a heavy pan, stirring continually until the sugar dissolves. Add chocolate.

Boil steadily, stirring, until a teaspoonful of fudge dropped into cold water forms a soft ball.

CHECK ALL ingredient labels EVERY TIME YOU BUY

Remove from the heat and plunge the pan in cold water to stop the cooking. Leave for 1-2 minutes, then beat with a wooden spoon until grainy, not glossy.

Pour into a buttered 30cm x 18cm (12"x7") shallow tin. Cool until nearly set and cut into squares.

Remove from tin and serve.

Lemon poppy seed cake

6 servings

grated rind of 2 lemons
65ml (4 tblsp) lemon juice
120g (4 oz) brown rice flour
100g (3½ oz) potato flour
100g (3½ oz) ground almonds
225g (8 oz) sugar
4 tblsp poppy seeds
3 tsp baking powder
1 tsp bicarbonate of soda
1 tsp xanthan gum
1 egg
120g (4 oz) silken tofu
125ml (4 fl oz, ½ US cup) milk
75ml (3 fl oz, $\frac{1}{3}$ US cup) oil
4 tsp tahini
2 tsp vanilla extract

Preheat oven to 180°C (350°F, gas mark 4).

Mix dry ingredients together with lemon rind.

Beat all wet ingredients together and add to dry ingredients. Mix well.

Pour into a greased and lined 20cm (8") cake tin.

Bake for 45 minutes to 1 hour until a knife comes out clean.

Decorate with lemon icing and top with poppy seeds.

CHECK ALL ingredient labels EVERY TIME YOU BUY

Coconut mountains

Makes 16 cakes

190ml (6 oz) can condensed milk
250g (8 oz) desiccated coconut
½ tsp vanilla essence
three or four different food colors

Preheat oven to 170°C (325°F, gas mark 3).

Mix coconut, milk and vanilla essence together. Divide into four portions and color three or four of them with different colors (one can be left white).

Lay sheets of rice paper or greased foil on baking sheets. Form the mixture into four pyramids of each color, each about 2.5cm (1") apart on the paper.

Bake for 15 minutes or until pale golden. Peel off foil if used or cut round if using rice paper. Cool on a wire rack.

Oatmeal raisin cookies

15 cookies

250g (9 oz) rice flour
150g (5 oz) potato flour
75g (2½ oz) arrowroot
1 tsp xanthan gum
180g (6 oz) butter, softened
150g (5 oz) white sugar
125g (4 oz) light brown sugar
2 eggs
1 tsp vanilla essence
200g (6½ oz) gluten free flour
1 tsp bicarbonate of soda
¾ tsp cinnamon
½ tsp salt
200g (6½ oz) rolled oats
200g (6½ oz) raisins

Preheat oven to 190°C (375°F, gas mark 5).

In a large bowl, cream together the butter and sugar

CHECK ALL ingredient labels EVERY TIME YOU BUY

until smooth. Beat in the eggs and vanilla, mixing until fluffy.

Stir together flour, bicarbonate of soda, cinnamon and salt. Gradually beat into the mixture.

Stir in the oats and raisins.

Place teaspoonsful onto a baking sheet, leaving room for them to spread a little.

Bake for 8-10 minutes until golden brown.

Transfer to a rack and allow to cool.

Sponge sandwich
Makes a 20cm cake

120g (4 oz) potato flour
60g (2 oz) rice flour
6 eggs, separated
6 oz caster sugar
1 tsp vanilla extract

Preheat oven to 180°C, (350°F, gas mark 4).

Whip yolks and sugar together until the mixture resembles mayonnaise. Add vanilla and a generous tablespoonful of egg whites.

Whisk remaining egg whites very stiff. Fold in the egg yolk mixture. Sieve flours together and fold in.

Turn into 2 prepared loose bottomed 20cm (8") cake tins.

Bake for about 30 minutes until cakes have shrunk around the sides of the tin.

Turn out, cool on a wire tray and sandwich with whipped cream, jam or both. Will freeze for 3 months.

CHECK ALL ingredient labels EVERY TIME YOU BUY

Caramel mud cake

12 servings

250g (9 oz) unsalted butter, chopped
225g (8 oz) white chocolate, chopped
400g (13 oz) brown sugar
375ml (12 fl oz, 1½ US cups) water
1 tsp vanilla extract
4 eggs, lightly beaten
275g (10 oz) gluten free flour
1½ tsp baking powder
1 tsp bicarbonate of soda

Frosting:
100g (3½ oz) butter, chopped
175g (6 oz) brown sugar
75ml (3 fl oz, $\frac{1}{3}$ US cup) milk
375g (13 oz) icing sugar

Preheat oven to 150°C (300°F, gas mark 2).

Grease and line the base and sides of a deep 22 cm (9") diameter round cake tin, bringing the paper 5 cm (2") above the sides of the tin.

Combine butter, chocolate, sugar and warm water in a medium saucepan, whisking over a low heat until the chocolate is melted and the sugar is dissolved.

Transfer mixture to a large bowl, leave to cool for 15 minutes.

Whisk in vanilla and eggs, then the flour mixture. Pour into the prepared cake tin.

Bake for about 2 hours. Cover cake loosely with foil if it starts to go too brown.

Cool the cake in the tin covered with a clean tea towel.

The cake can be frozen at this point, or iced with frosting.

If you are icing the cake, melt the butter in a small pan while the cake is cooling, stir in the brown sugar and

CHECK ALL ingredient labels EVERY TIME YOU BUY

milk, and bring to the boil.

Cook, stirring, for about 3 minutes. Leave to cool.

Add enough sifted icing sugar mixture to give a spreading consistency and stir until smooth.

Spread the cold cake with the frosting. Store in an airtight container at room temperature.

Stuffed dates
500g (1 lb) fresh or dried dates
180g (6 oz) marzipan
Icing sugar to coat (optional)

Slit each date along one long side and prise out the stone carefully, so as not to spoil the shape of the fruit.

Roll teaspoonfuls of marzipan into the same sort of shape as the removed stones. Stuff each date and roll in icing sugar.

Store in an airtight container in a cool place.

CHECK ALL ingredient labels EVERY TIME YOU BUY

TERRINES AND PATÉ

Blue cheese terrine

6 Servings

150ml (¼ UK pint, ⅝ US cup) sour cream
150ml (¼ UK pint, ⅝ US cup) mayonnaise
125g (4 oz) blue cheese, crumbled (Stilton is best)
1 tsp garlic powder or minced fresh cloves
½ tsp black pepper or ground peppercorns

Mix all ingredients together. Refrigerate for a few hours to let the flavors combine a little.

Serve.

This will keep in the fridge for 5 days to a week so if you don't think you can use it in that time halve the ingredients and make a smaller batch. It is also very chunky. If you want it less chunky reduce the amount of cheese.

Brawn

6-8 Servings

half a pig's head, cut in 2 or 3 pieces
2 pig's trotters
salt
2 medium onions, quartered
1 large carrot sliced
2 bay leaves
6 peppercorns
6 cloves
1 level tsp salt
pepper

Wash pig's head thoroughly, put in a large bowl with the trotters. Cover with water, add a handful of salt and leave to soak overnight.

Drain and put into a large pan or pressure cooker. Cover with water and bring to the boil, removing scum.

Add onion, carrot, bay leaves, peppercorns and cloves.

CHECK ALL ingredient labels EVERY TIME YOU BUY

Cover and simmer for 2½ hours, or pressure cook under high pressure for 20 minutes, until tender.

Remove meat from pan, separate from skin and bones. Cut the meat into pieces and set aside.

Return bones to the pan, add salt and boil rapidly until the liquid is reduced to about 450ml (¾ pint). Strain and leave to cool.

Skim fat from the surface of the stock. Mix liquid with meat and season to taste. Transfer to a large (1½lb) loaf tin and leave in the refrigerator to set.

To serve, turn out and slice. Serve with watercress or chicory salad.

Smoked haddock paté
4 Servings

350g (¾ lb) smoked haddock
275ml (½ UK pint, 1¼ US cups) milk
300g (10 oz) unsalted butter, melted
1 lemon, halved
black pepper
1 level tsp chopped fresh parsley

Poach fish in milk until just cooked, about 10 minutes. Drain. Remove all skin and bone.

Put fish into blender with melted butter. Add the juice of half a lemon and pepper to taste.

Blend until smooth. Turn into a bowl or individual serving dishes. Chill until firm.

Garnish with parsley and slices of lemon. Serve with Corn Thins or rice cakes.

CHECK ALL ingredient labels EVERY TIME YOU BUY

Liver paté

8 Servings

250g (½ lb) pigs' liver
250g (½ lb) chicken livers
125g (¼ lb) streaky bacon
1 level tsp mustard powder
1 onion, chopped
1 clove garlic, crushed
1 level tsp salt
pepper
1 egg, beaten
60g (2 oz) butter, melted

Preheat oven to 150°C (300°F, gas mark 2).

Slice up the pigs liver and chicken livers and the bacon. Mix with the other ingredients.

Put half the mixture into the blender and blend until smooth. Transfer to a mixing bowl. Blend the second half a little rougher and mix in.

Turn into a small (1lb) oiled loaf tin, cover with greaseproof and foil. Stand in a baking tray half full of water.

Bake for 2 hours. Remove from oven and cool.

Turn out, chill, and serve with toast.

Can be frozen for up to 1 month: thaw overnight in the refrigerator or for 3 hours at room temperature.

CHECK ALL ingredient labels EVERY TIME YOU BUY

RECIPES KIDS LOVE

Farmhouse paté
Servings vary

375g (¾ lb) belly pork rashers
500g (1 lb) lean stewing beef
250g (½ lb) pigs' liver
1 small onion, chopped finely
2 level tsp salt
½ tsp pepper
2 tblsp wine vinegar
1 tblsp brandy or white Vermouth
1 level tsp dried basil
1 egg, beaten
2 bay leaves

Preheat oven to 180°C (350°F, gas mark 4).

Trim meat and cut into pieces, then mince with a medium cutter, or chop as small as you can. Season with salt, pepper, vinegar and brandy. Mix well and leave to stand for 2 hours.

Add egg, onion and basil to the mixed meat and mix well. Spoon into a large (2 lb) loaf tin, smoothing the surface. Top with bay leaves.

Set in a roasting tin and add water to half-way up the sides. Bake for 2½-3 hours.

Remove from oven and leave to cool. When cool, place a weight on top and refrigerate.

CHECK ALL ingredient labels EVERY TIME YOU BUY

Stuffed duck

10 Servings

2.5 kg (5 lb) duck, boned by the butcher
125g (4 oz) cooked rice
175g (6 oz) cooked Morello (sour) cherries, stoned, drained and chopped
60g (2 oz) pistachio nuts, chopped
2 medium onions, chopped and lightly fried
2 eggs, beaten
1 level tsp dried tarragon
1 level tsp salt
pepper
2 tblsp clear honey

Preheat oven to 200°C (400 °F, gas mark 6).

Wash and dry duck.

Mix all the other ingredients except the honey together. Use to stuff duck, pushing into corners and folding the skin round to form a natural shape.

Sew up.

Prick well all over with a large needle.

Place on a rack in a roasting tin and bake for 1 hour, basting occasionally.

Brush honey over duck and bake for a further 30 minutes, basting frequently.

Remove from the oven, cool, and chill until firm.

Carve into slices. Serve with lettuce and watercress.

CHECK ALL ingredient labels EVERY TIME YOU BUY

SALADS: MAIN COURSE SALADS

Hot Chinese style chicken salad
2 Servings

2 chicken breasts, cooked with desired seasoning
2 large bowls of lettuce
Choice of: tomatoes, crumbled bacon, hot peppers,
    slivered almonds
Grated cheese

Dressing:
150ml (¼ UK pint, $\frac{5}{8}$ US cup) oil
75ml (3 fl oz, $\frac{1}{3}$ US cup) cider vinegar
1 tblsp gluten free soy sauce
2 tsp sugar
a little powdered ginger
a little garlic salt
pepper

Prepare salad, dividing evenly between two plates or
bowls.

Bring dressing ingredients to the boil in a pan and stir
with whisk. Once all ingredients are well-blended, pour
over salads.

Kentucky Derby salad
1 Serving

iceberg lettuce
1 tblsp cider vinegar
4 strips bacon
half an onion
brown sugar
2 tblsp sesame oil

Grill bacon very crisp, drain well.

Shred lettuce, dice or slice the onions, crunch up bacon,
mix together.

Mix sesame oil with vinegar and brown sugar to taste.
Pour over salad.

CHECK ALL ingredient labels EVERY TIME YOU BUY

Black and blue salad

4 Servings

150ml (¼ UK pint, ⅝ US cups) double (heavy) cream
2 tblsp mayonnaise
170g (6 oz) blue cheese (Stilton is best)
1 tblsp vinegar (optional)
2 butterhead (soft) lettuces
170g (6 oz) cold cooked beef, thinly sliced
8 cherry tomatoes, cut in half

Beat the cream and mayonnaise together in a small mixing bowl. Crumble half the blue cheese into the mixture (reserving the other half for a garnish) and stir a few times. Add a drizzle of the vinegar if it is too thick.

Chill for at least two hours. (The longer it chills, the more intense the flavor becomes.)

Cut the butterhead lettuce in wedges (or tear into pieces if you prefer) and place on four salad plates.

Pour the blue cheese dressing over the lettuce. Arrange strips of the cold beef and four cherry tomato halves over the lettuce. Sprinkle the reserved blue cheese on top.

Season with freshly ground pepper and serve immediately.

Spicy chicken taco style salad

4 Servings

4 chicken breasts
2 tblsp olive oil
2 tsp cumin seed
1-2 tsp chilli powder
1 can tomatoes with green chillis (jalapenos)
1 large yellow onion, diced
salt and pepper
1 iceberg lettuce
1 can black olives
60g (2 oz) grated cheddar cheese
1 carton sour cream

CHECK ALL ingredient labels EVERY TIME YOU BUY

Guacamole (optional)

Poach the chicken breasts in a little stock or water, remove and use a fork to shred.

In a large skillet, heat olive oil over a medium heat and use to sautée about a quarter of the onions with the cumin and chilli powder.

Stir in the shredded chicken and chopped tomatoes with chillis, along with the juice. Simmer for approximately 20 minutes, stirring occasionally.

Meanwhile, shred lettuce and place in bowls. When chicken mixture is done, pile on top of the lettuce and cover with guacamole if used, sour cream, the remaining onions, olives and cheese.

Serve with Homemade Salsa.

Cajun chicken Caesar salad
1 Serving

1 large chicken breast
cajun spice or cayenne pepper to taste
2 tblsp gluten free hot sauce
Half a large cos lettuce
2 tblsp gluten free Caesar dressing
2 tblsp parmesan cheese

Season the chicken breast with the spices.

Grill or chargrill chicken until cooked through, then cut into 2cm (1 inch) cubes, add hot sauce and mix well. Set aside.

Break lettuce into small pieces, mix with dressing and cheese and plate up. Top with chicken.

Sprinkle with more parmesan cheese if desired.

Use cayenne if you like it really hot and spicy. Cajun spice will make it a little milder.

CHECK ALL ingredient labels EVERY TIME YOU BUY

Zesty shrimp salad
3 Servings

500g (1 lb) shrimps or prawns
1 small head of lettuce
half a medium cucumber
1 green pepper
60ml (2 fl oz, ¼ US cup) GF Italian salad dressing

Bring 2 pints of water to the boil and drop shrimps in boiling water for 5 to 7 minutes. Drain and leave to cool.

When shrimps are cool, peel and mix into salad dressing.

Cut the other ingredients into bite size pieces, add the shrimps and mix well.

Seven layer salad
lettuce
sliced hard boiled eggs
chopped onion
sliced olives
crumbled bacon
mayonnaise
grated cheese

Build up in layers in single serving size or family size. Can be made ahead and refrigerated.

Curried prawn salad
2 Servings

about a third of a lettuce
4 radishes, chopped
3 spring (green) onions, finely chopped
half a green pepper, chopped (optional)
2 tblsp butter
250g (½ lb) cooked prawns
1 clove garlic
pepper
3 tblsp mayonnaise
1 tsp curry powder

Put about 2 tblsp butter and 250g cooked prawns in a

CHECK ALL ingredient labels EVERY TIME YOU BUY

medium glass bowl. Cover. Microwave 1 minute till butter is melted and prawns are medium hot.

Stir in 1 clove crushed garlic and a small amount of pepper.

In a separate small bowl combine 3 large tblsp of mayonnaise and 1 tsp curry powder.

Pour juice from prawns into mayonnaise and combine. Put prawns on top of salad. Pour dressing on salad.

Prawn egg salad
2 Servings

2 hard boiled eggs
2 tblsp mayonnaise
250g (½ lb) frozen prawns

Drop frozen prawns into boiling water for 1 min then drain.

Chop boiled eggs into bowl, add mayonnaise and mix well. Add prawns. Mix and chill.

Good on a bed of chopped spinach, or just by itself.

Sante Fe beef and hot pepper salad
8 Servings

150ml (¼ UK pint, ⅝ US cups) pitted ripe olives
250g (½ lb) lettuce, torn up
250g (½ lb) roast beef, cut into fine strips
125g (¼ lb) hot pepper cheese
2 medium tomatoes, cut into thin wedges
2 thin onion slices, separated into rings

Dressing:
125ml (4 fl oz, ½ US cup) gluten free salsa
125ml (4 fl oz, ½ US cup) sour cream
½ tsp chilli powder

Stir together salsa, sour cream and chilli powder in a small bowl. Mix well.

Combine all salad ingredients in large bowl, toss lightly. Serve with dressing.

CHECK ALL ingredient labels EVERY TIME YOU BUY

RECIPES KIDS LOVE

Bacon and egg salad

4 Servings

8 hard boiled eggs
275ml (½ UK pint, 1¼ US cups) mayonnaise
250g (½ lb) bacon rashers
250g (½ lb) hot pepper cheese
3 tblsp chives
4 thin radishes
1 head lettuce
1 avocado

Fry bacon until crisp, drain well and crumble.

Dice eggs, avocado and cheese. Slice radishes and tear lettuce into small pieces. Mix with bacon and mayonnaise.

Chop chives and sprinkle over salad before serving.

Grilled chicken salad

6 Servings

60ml (2 fl oz, ¼ US cup) gluten free dark soy sauce
60ml (2 fl oz, ¼ US cup) olive oil
1 kg (2 lb) skinless boneless chicken breast, diced
1 clove garlic, crushed
2 tblsp gluten free light soy sauce
2 cups lettuce
1 large tomato
1 medium cucumber
Half a red onion
black pepper, to taste
balsamic vinegar, to taste

Heat oil in a non-stick frying pan. Sauté chicken with garlic until just starting to turn golden brown.

Add dark soy sauce. Simmer over a low heat for about 5 to 10 minutes. The oil will float a little to the top. That's okay.

Make salad with the remaining items. Sprinkle with black

CHECK ALL ingredient labels EVERY TIME YOU BUY

pepper.

When salad is ready, pour the hot mixture of chicken, oil and soy sauce onto the salad.

Add balsamic vinegar to taste and toss.

Warm turkey salad

1-2 Servings

250g (½ lb) minced turkey
a good handful of mixed salad leaves
1 tomato
4 or 5 Kalamata olives
salt and pepper
1-2 tblsp olive oil
1 clove crushed garlic
a few leaves of finely chopped fresh basil
Dice the tomato and place in a small bowl. Add chopped olives, olive oil, garlic, basil, and salt and pepper to taste.

Brown the turkey mince in a saucepan. Add the tomato mix to the turkey and mix together.

Serve over a bed of mixed salad leaves.

Philly cheese steak salad

2 Servings

4 thin steaks, cut into strips
1 onion, sliced
1 green pepper, sliced
4 slices Provolone cheese
Lettuce
6 cherry tomatoes, quartered
2 tblsp mayonnaise
1 tblsp salad oil

Brown onion and green pepper in a little oil in skillet. Add steak strips and cook until done.

Add slices of Provolone cheese and cook for a few seconds until the cheese starts to melt. Serve on a bed of lettuce topped with tomatoes and mayonnaise.

CHECK ALL ingredient labels EVERY TIME YOU BUY

Bacon cheeseburger salad

4 Servings

250g (8 oz) lean minced beef
4 rashers of streaky bacon
half a crisp lettuce
1 spring (green) onion
1 medium tomato
1-2 tblsp mayonnaise
30g (1 oz) cheddar cheese, grated

Cook minced beef in salted water, breaking it up as it cooks. Drain well.

Fry bacon until crisp, drain well and crumble. Chop lettuce, onion and tomato.

Stir mayonnaise into lettuce, onion and tomato until evenly coated. Stir in beef, bacon and cheese. Serve with gluten free panbread.

Instant prawn salad

1 Serving

1 carton gluten free prawn cocktail
half a cucumber
lettuce to taste
A selection of: a small slice of white cabbage, 1 tblsp
    sultanas, 1-2 sticks celery, 2 or 3 cherry tomatoes, 2
    spring (green) onions, 1 tblsp drained canned
    sweetcorn
black pepper

Shred lettuce. Cut the cucumber into quarters lengthwise, then cut each quarter into small chunks. Cut celery into similar sized pieces. Cut tomatoes in half. Shred cabbage. Separate sultanas, wash and remove any stalks. Chop spring (green) onions or leave whole.

Mix vegetables and fruit together and place on a plate. Season with pepper.

Top with prawn cocktail and a little more pepper, if liked. Serve.

CHECK ALL ingredient labels EVERY TIME YOU BUY

Warm chicken and bacon club salad
4-6 Servings

4 boneless skinless chicken breasts
275ml (½ UK pint, 1¼ US cups) mayonnaise
6 rashers bacon
250g (½ lb) grated cheddar cheese
A few chopped black olives to garnish(optional)

Preheat oven to 150°C (300°F, gas mark 2).

Poach chicken breasts in a little stock for about 15 minutes (make sure the water is bubbling the whole time). Remove from stock and dice.

Cook bacon until crisp, then crumble.

Mix all the ingredients together and spread into a 20cm (8") cake pan.

Bake for about 15 minutes.

Serve on top of a bed of lettuce.

Top with black olives if you like.

Turkey and ham salad
2 Servings

1 small cauliflower
1 cucumber, cut into bite-sized pieces
3 cherry tomatoes, halved
1 thick slice ham, diced
1 thick slice turkey, diced
Mayonnaise
Salt and pepper

Cook the cauliflower for about 10 minutes until tender but not soft. Drain and cut into bite sized pieces.

Add the cucumber, tomatoes, ham and turkey. Mix with mayonnaise and add salt and pepper.

Chill.

CHECK ALL ingredient labels EVERY TIME YOU BUY

BLT salad
4 Servings

7 rashers bacon, cooked crisp, drained and crumbled
250g (9 oz, 1 US cup) chopped lettuce
1 tblsp chopped onion
half a medium tomato, chopped
1 tblsp mayonnaise

Stir mayonnaise into lettuce, onion and tomato until evenly coated.

Add bacon and mix well.

CHECK ALL ingredient labels EVERY TIME YOU BUY

SALADS: MAIN COURSE - VEGETARIAN

Mexican egg salad

4 Servings

6 large hard boiled eggs
1 small red pepper, chopped
3 ounce can green chilli (jalapeno) peppers, finely
  chopped
2 tblsp mayonnaise
1 tsp American mustard
a pinch of cayenne pepper

Quarter eggs, mix with the other ingredients and serve.

Great served with roasted red peppers.

Waldorf salad

4 Servings

500g jicama or water chestnuts, peeled and cubed
2 tblsp lemon juice
4 or 5 strawberries
2 sticks celery, sliced
150ml (¼ pint) mayonnaise, more or less to taste
2 tsp sugar
3 tblsp slivered almonds
2 tblsp blue cheese, crumbled (optional)
4 cups cos lettuce, shredded

Toss jicama or water chestnut cubes with lemon juice
and leave to stand for 5 minutes.

Cut strawberries into quarters and mix in, along with the
remaining ingredients, except lettuce.

Refrigerate for at least half an hour before serving.

Divide lettuce among 4 plates and spoon salad over the
top.

CHECK ALL ingredient labels EVERY TIME YOU BUY

Pecan and gorgonzola salad

1 Serving

3-4 lettuce leaves
60g (2 oz) gorgonzola cheese
60g (2 oz) pecan pieces
30g (1 oz) butter
olive oil
balsamic vinegar
salt and pepper
half a dessert pear, chopped (optional)

Melt butter and add pecan pieces. Toast carefully, stirring continuously. Be careful because the pecans will burn before the butter.

Cut gorgonzola into small cubes. Mix with toasted pecans and the other ingredients, except lettuce and vinegar.

Serve on a bed of lettuce, with a drizzle of balsamic vinegar.

Butter bean (lima bean) salad

4 Servings

1 lettuce heart
250g (½ lb) cooked butter (lima) beans
250g (½ lb) cooked peas
1 sliced onion
vinaigrette dressing
salt

Line bowl with crisped, salted lettuce. Drain beans and peas, and mix with dressing and sliced onion. Pour on top of the lettuce and serve.

CHECK ALL ingredient labels EVERY TIME YOU BUY

RECIPES KIDS LOVE

Cauliflower and egg salad
4 Servings

1 cauliflower
2 hard boiled eggs
1 onion
1 stick celery
75ml (3 fl oz, $\frac{1}{3}$ US cup) mayonnaise
½ tsp mustard powder
½-1 tsp seasoned rice vinegar
salt and pepper
1 tblsp chopped fresh dill (optional)
1 chopped dill pickle (optional)

Break cauliflower into florets and cook in boiling salted water until just cooked, but still crisp - about 10 minutes. Drain and allow to cool for a few minutes while preparing the other ingredients.

Chop eggs, onion, celery and dill pickle, if used. Mix with mayonnaise, mustard, vinegar and seasoning to taste. Stir in cauliflower, making sure it is well coated with the sauce.

Sprinkle with chopped dill, if used. Serve chilled.

CHECK ALL ingredient labels EVERY TIME YOU BUY

Monaco salad

1 Serving

half a cos lettuce
half a head of pak choi
4-5 endive leaves
250g (½ lb) spinach, stems removed
1 slice of cup red cabbage
one third of a cucumber
2 sticks celery
125g (¼ lb) mushrooms
1 small jicama or carrot, peeled
1 tsp poppy seeds
275ml (½ UK pint, 1¼ US cups) vinaigrette dressing

Shred lettuce, pak choi, spinach and endive coarsely and cabbage finely. Slice cucumber, celery and mushrooms. Grate jicama or carrot.

Mix vegetables together, pour over dressing and mix again. Sprinkle with poppy seeds before serving.

SALADS: SIDE SALADS
(MOSTLY VEGETARIAN)

Achar timun (Malaysian cucumber salad) (contains prawns)
4 Servings

1 small cucumber
1 tblsp cooked prawns or shrimps
125ml (4 fl oz, ½ US cup) thick coconut milk
1 small sliced onion
1 chopped red chilli (jalapeno)
little anchovy essence
salt

Wash and peel cucumber and cut into 5cm (2 in) lengths. With a small knife cut thinly round and round towards the centre. Roll up the strip and thinly slice.

Wash and pound the prawns.

Mix all the ingredients together, chill and serve.

Cauliflower-broccoli salad
16 Servings

1 large cauliflower
1 large bunch broccoli
1 small onion (or 4 spring (green) onions)
1 small packet frozen peas
570ml (1 UK pint, 2½ US cups) mayonnaise
275ml (½ UK pint, 1¼ US cups) sour cream
1 tsp garlic powder

Defrost peas and drain well.

Mix mayonnaise, sour cream and garlic powder in a small bowl.

Break cauliflower and broccoli into bite sized florets. Add onion and mix together. Stir into sauce and mix well.

Stir in peas. Refrigerate for at least 4 hours or overnight before serving.

CHECK ALL ingredient labels EVERY TIME YOU BUY

Pickled mushroom salad

4 Servings

570ml (1 UK pint, 2½ US cups) pickled mushrooms
75ml (3 fl oz, $\frac{1}{3}$ US cup) sour cream
black pepper
half an onion, chopped

Drain pickled mushrooms and slice, add chopped onion and mix with sour cream.

flavor with pepper.

Mushroom salad

6 Servings

500g (1 lb) mushrooms, sliced
1 tsp salt
3 tblsp olive oil
juice of half a lemon
275ml (½ UK pint, 1¼ US cups) water
1 bay leaf
1 sprig thyme
6 black peppercorns, crushed
6 coriander seeds, crushed
3 tomatoes, skinned and chopped
1 clove garlic, crushed

Place all ingredients in a heavy saucepan. Bring to the boil, cover and turn heat right down.

Cook for 25 minutes, cool and drain.

Remove herbs. Arrange in dish and chill.

Italian cauliflower salad

6 Servings

1 cauliflower divided into florets
2 tblsp diced green pepper
2 tblsp diced onion
60ml (2 fl oz, ¼ US cup) water
3 tblsp gluten free Italian salad dressing
¼ tsp salt
a pinch of dried oregano

CHECK ALL ingredient labels EVERY TIME YOU BUY

a pinch of dried basil
a pinch of garlic powder

Combine all ingredients in pan. Cover and cook over medium heat, stirring once in a while till cauliflower is tender but still crisp, about 10 minutes. Chill thoroughly.

Mushroom and olive salad
6 Servings

150ml (¼ UK pint, ⅝ US cup) kalamata olives
150ml (¼ UK pint, ⅝ US cup) green olives
150ml (¼ UK pint, ⅝ US cup) black olives
1 yellow sweet pepper, diced
1 small jar pimientos
125g (¼ lb) button mushrooms, halved
275ml (½ UK pint, 1¼ US cups) gluten free Italian salad dressing
3 tblsp lemon juice
1 tsp freshly ground black pepper
2 cloves garlic, crushed
2 cups water
½ tsp salt

Use whole, pitted olives –or olive halves (not slices) as preferred.

Drain and rinse all ingredients.

Bring water, salt and lemon juice to the boil. Add mushrooms and boil for 3 minutes. Drain well.

Warm salad dressing, garlic and pepper to a low simmer, then remove from heat and allow to cool while you assemble the rest.

In a large dish, place olives, mushrooms, pimento and peppers. When dressing has cooled slightly, pour over and cover. Marinate for 2-3 days, stirring occasionally.

CHECK ALL ingredient labels EVERY TIME YOU BUY

German hot turnip salad (contains bacon)
2-4 Servings

1 large turnip
275ml (½ UK pint, 1¼ US cups) mayonnaise
3 tblsp white wine
2 tsp vinegar
½ tsp fresh dill
2 tsp sugar
¾ tsp salt
a pinch of pepper
bacon strips, cooked crisp and crushed
150ml (¼ UK pint, $\frac{5}{8}$ UK cup) bacon fat
2 tblsp onion

Cut turnip into cubes and boil in salted water until soft. Drain. Sauté onion in the reserved bacon fat.

Whisk mayonnaise, wine, vinegar, dill and seasonings together. (Makes about 2 cups of dressing. Use about ¼ to ½ cup per large turnip, storing remainder in a screw top jar in the refrigerator.) Use as much as required to dress turnip.

Add crushed bacon and onions.

Takeaway-style coleslaw
10 Servings

1 white cabbage, finely chopped, not shredded
60g (2 oz) chopped carrot, finely chopped
75g (2½ oz) caster sugar
½ tsp salt and a pinch of white pepper
30ml (1 fl oz, $\frac{1}{8}$ US cup) single cream
30ml (1 fl oz, $\frac{1}{8}$ US cup) whole milk
125ml (4 fl oz, ½ US cup) mayonnaise
60ml (2 fl oz, ¼ US cup) buttermilk
1½ tblsp white vinegar
2½ tblsp lemon juice

Be sure cabbage and carrots are chopped up into very fine pieces (about the size of rice.) If you have no food processor, cabbage and carrots may be chopped by

CHECK ALL ingredient labels EVERY TIME YOU BUY

adding small pieces of them to your blender with cold water and hitting the medium-low setting. Be sure to drain very well before proceeding.

Combine sugar, salt, pepper, cream, milk, mayonnaise, buttermilk, vinegar and lemon juice in a large bowl and beat until smooth.

Add the cabbage and carrots and mix well.

Cover and refrigerate for at least 2 hours before serving.

Guacamole
4-6 Servings

3-4 large ripe avocados (or 5-6 small)
1 medium red onion
2-3 firm red tomatoes
1 lime
2-3 fresh chillies (jalapenos)
Salt and pepper
2 tblsp chopped fresh coriander
1-2 cloves garlic, crushed and finely chopped (optional)

Chop the tomatoes into 1cm (¼") cubes and put in a colander to drain off excess juice.

Slice avocado lengthwise, and twist to separate the two halves. Using a sharp knife, cut the flesh inside into cubes, but don't cut through the skin. Scoop out the cubes of avocado and place in a suitable container for mashing.

Mash the avocado up a bit, but don't overdo it.

Remove the seeds from the jalapeno and chop it finely, along with the onion. Add to the mashed avocado, together with the juice from the lime and the garlic, if used. Season with salt and pepper and mix well.

Just before serving, stir in the chopped tomatoes, then pile back into the avocado shells.

CHECK ALL ingredient labels EVERY TIME YOU BUY

Fancy pea salad (contains bacon)
4-6 Servings

250g (½ lb) cooked peas
1 finely chopped onion
4 sticks celery, chopped
570ml (1 UK pint, 2½ US cups) torn up lettuce
275ml (½ UK pint, 1¼ US cups) mayonnaise
10 rashers bacon, cooked, drained and crumbled
60g (2 oz) grated Parmesan cheese

Toss peas, onion, celery, and lettuce with mayonnaise in a serving bowl. Sprinkle bacon and Parmesan cheese on top. Cover. Refrigerate overnight before serving.

Italian mushroom salad
2 Servings

3 tblsp gluten free Italian salad dressing
1 tblsp Parmesan cheese
250g (½ lb) mushrooms, thinly sliced

Mix dressing and cheese.

Stir in mushrooms. Chill for several hours.

Easy egg plant salad
4 servings

1 large aubergine (eggplant)
1 large onion
1 can pitted black olives
1 small jar Spanish olives
60ml (2 fl oz, ¼ US cups) cider vinegar (or to taste)
1 litre (1¾ UK pints, 4½ US cups) gluten free tomato
   sauce
cayenne pepper *or* black pepper to taste

Preheat oven to 170°C (325°F, gas mark 3).

Cut aubergine and onion into 1cm (½") cubes and olives into small pieces. Put into an ovenproof dish.

Add vinegar to chopped ingredients. Mix well.

CHECK ALL ingredient labels EVERY TIME YOU BUY

Mix in the tomato sauce and cayenne or black pepper to taste (½ tsp cayenne is hot).

Bake for 1 hour. Remove from oven and leave to cool.

When cold, stir and refrigerate before serving.

Broccoli, olive and egg salad
4 Servings

1 pack fresh broccoli, cut into florets
3 hard boiled eggs, quartered
150ml (¼ UK pint, ⅝ US cup) green olives, drained
half a large red onion, chopped
Mayonnaise
Salt and black pepper
Paprika to garnish

Mix everything together and coat well with mayonnaise. Dust lightly with paprika. Chill and serve.

Peanut coleslaw
8 Servings

1 medium head white cabbage
90g (3 oz) salted peanuts
275ml (½ UK pint, 1¼ US cups) sour cream
150ml (¼ UK pint, ⅝ US cup) mayonnaise
a pinch of sugar

In a food processor chop the cabbage semi-fine.

Remove and process almost all the peanuts until chopped coarsely (be careful not to process too long or you'll have peanut butter).

Mix the sour cream, mayonnaise and sugar to taste, then mix with cabbage and chopped and whole peanuts.

Leave to stand for a few hours in the fridge to blend flavors.

CHECK ALL ingredient labels EVERY TIME YOU BUY

Sesame coleslaw
8-10 Servings

½ cup sesame seeds
½ cup slivered almonds
2 tblsp butter
1 head cabbage, shredded
4 spring (green) onions, chopped

Dressing:
1/3 cup red wine vinegar
½ cup olive oil
8 tsp sugar
2 tsp salt
¼ tsp pepper

Sauté sesame seeds and almonds in butter. Add to cabbage and spring (green) onions. Refrigerate.

Mix dressing and pour over salad.

Alu raita (Pakistan spiced potato salad)
4 Servings

3-4 large potatoes
2 cups dahi
½ tsp toasted cumin seeds
salt and pepper
2 tblsp chopped coriander
chilli powder to taste
2-3 medium tomatoes
few sprigs coriander to garnish

Boil potatoes in their skins until tender. Cool, peel and slice fairly thinly.

Beat dahi until smooth, add cumin seeds, salt, pepper, coriander and chilli.

Drop the tomatoes alternately into boiling and iced water to loosen their skins, peel and slice, discarding the seeds and core.

Mix with the potatoes carefully and add dahi mixture.

Chill and garnish with coriander sprigs to serve.

CHECK ALL ingredient labels EVERY TIME YOU BUY

Thanthat (Burmese cucumber salad)
4-6 Servings

3 medium cucumbers
3 tblsp vinegar
salt
150ml (¼ UK pint, $\frac{5}{8}$ US cup) sesame oil
1 large finely chopped onion
20 cloves garlic, roughly chopped
1 tsp turmeric
2 tblsp Kaey-Garu or sesame seeds

Peel cucumbers, remove seeds and cut into strips about 2cm long. Put into enough boiling water to cover, adding vinegar. Bring back to the boil, cook until transparent, drain and sprinkle lightly with salt.

Heat oil and fry onion until golden, remove and fry garlic in the same way, remove and keep separate.

Add turmeric, salt and half the sesame seeds and fry for a few minutes until fragrant. Remove from heat and cool.

Mix this dressing with the cucumber, pile onto a dish and garnish with remaining sesame seeds.

Surround with fried onion and garlic.

If there is too much dressing, the remainder can be served separately.

CHECK ALL ingredient labels EVERY TIME YOU BUY

Oriental salad

8 Servings

250-500g (½-1 lb) white cabbage, finely shredded
250g (½ lb) red cabbage, finely shredded
6 spring (green) onions, sliced thin
4 tsp toasted sesame seeds
Oriental Dressing:
3-4 tblsp sesame oil
6 tblsp red wine vinegar
1-2 tsp sugar
pepper

Prepare salad greens, onions and sesame seeds and layer in a glass bowl. Cover and chill.

Mix all dressing ingredients and leavestand at room temperature for 30 minutes.

Just before serving, add dressing to salad and toss.

CHECK ALL ingredient labels EVERY TIME YOU BUY

RECIPES KIDS LOVE

Chunky tomato salad
1-2 Servings

250g (½ lb) fresh tomatoes
60g (2 oz,) spring (green) onions
125g (¼ lb) mushrooms
1 tblsp olive oil
1 tblsp vinegar
1 tblsp water
1 tsp dried basil
a pinch of dried oregano
½ tsp sugar
salt and pepper to taste

Cut tomatoes into 2cm (1") chunks. Slice onions and mushrooms.

In a large bowl mix oil, vinegar, water, herbs and seasoning. Mix well and add chopped ingredients. Stir gently until spices are evenly spread throughout. Chill overnight.

Pineapple slaw
4 Servings

a large slice of white cabbage, finely shredded
half a tin crushed pineapple in juice, drained
60g (2 oz) green peppers, finely diced
2 tblsp mayonnaise
1 onion, finely diced
1 tsp sugar
¼ tsp celery seed
salt and pepper

Combine pineapple and vegetables. Mix well.

Mix the rest of the ingredients together. Spoon over salad.

Stir well. Chill. Stir again just before serving.

CHECK ALL ingredient labels EVERY TIME YOU BUY

Classic coleslaw

1 Serving

A medium slice of white cabbage
half a carrot
half an onion (optional)
2 tblsp of mayonnaise
2 tsp white distilled vinegar
salt and pepper to taste

Shred cabbage, carrot and onion finely and mix with other ingredients.

Double cranberry salad

8 Servings

570ml (1 UK pint, 2½ US cups) Iced Botanicals
   (Cranberry-Raspberry)
1 large packet cranberry or raspberry jelly
2 sticks chopped celery
90g (3 oz) chopped pecans
250g (9 oz) cottage cheese
30ml (1 fl oz, $\frac{1}{8}$ US cup) mayonnaise

Bring Botanicals to the boil. Stir in jelly mix until dissolved. Chill until partially set. Pour half into a 750ml glass dish.

Stir half the celery and nuts into dish. Chill until firm.

Mix mayonnaise and cottage cheese together and pile on top of the contents of the dish. Flatten out. Warm the remaining jelly in the microwave until it is pourable and pour over the cottage cheese.

Chill until firm. Cut into 8 portions.

CHECK ALL ingredient labels EVERY TIME YOU BUY

Potato pickle salad

6 Servings

750g (1½ lb) new potatoes, boiled
1 large sweet-sour gherkin (dill pickle)
 or 2 tblsp pickled capers
4 tblsp mayonnaise
2-3 spring (green) onions

This is particularly tasty if made when the potatoes are still fairly warm.

Cut potatoes into chunks about 2.5cm (1") across.

Chop gherkin (or capers) and onions fairly small.

Stir gherkin or caper mixture into the mayonnaise in a large bowl. Add in the potatoes and stir to completely coat them with the mayonnaise.

Serve immediately.

CHECK ALL ingredient labels EVERY TIME YOU BUY

SALADS: DRESSINGS AND DIPS

Caesar salad dressing
Makes 300 ml

275ml (½ UK pint, 1¼ US cups) mayonnaise
1 egg yolk
60g (2 oz) grated parmesan cheese
2 tblsp water
2 tblsp olive oil
1½ tblsp lemon juice
1 tblsp anchovy paste
2 cloves garlic, crushed
2 tsp sugar
½ tsp coarsely ground pepper
¼ tsp salt
¼ tsp dried parsley, powdered

Combine all ingredients in a medium bowl and beat with an electric mixer for about 1 minute.

Cover and chill for several hours to develop the flavors.

Cheesy herb dressing
Makes 150 ml

150ml (¼ UK pint, ⅝ US cup) gluten free yogurt
1 tblsp olive oil
1 tblsp grated Parmesan cheese
¼ tsp dried basil
1 tblsp dried parsley
1½ tsp lemon juice
¼ tsp garlic powder

Combine all ingredients and mix well. Chill overnight.

Creamy Italian dressing
Makes 250 ml

150ml (¼ UK pint, ⅝ US cup) plain gluten free yogurt
60ml (2 fl oz, ¼ US cup) mayonnaise
2 tblsp double (heavy) cream

CHECK ALL ingredient labels EVERY TIME YOU BUY

1 tblsp red wine vinegar
½ tsp dried oregano
½ tsp dried basil
½ tsp sugar
a pinch of garlic powder
salt and pepper

Combine all and mix well. Chill several hours or overnight.

Blue cheese dressing
Makes 1 litre

500ml (¾ UK pint, 2 US cups) mayonnaise
125ml (4 fl oz, ½ US cup) sour cream
340g (11½ oz) soft blue cheese
garlic powder to taste
a dash of vinegar
finely chopped onion

Combine all ingredients in a blender until smooth.

Ginger salad dressing
6 Servings

60g (2 oz) chopped onion
60ml (2 fl oz, ¼ US cup) peanut oil
2 tblsp rice wine vinegar
2 tblsp water
1 tblsp chopped ginger root
1 tblsp chopped celery
1 tblsp gluten free soy sauce
1½ tsp tomato paste
1½ tsp sugar
1 tsp lemon juice
salt and pepper

Combine all ingredients. Process until almost smooth.

May be kept refrigerated up to one week.

CHECK ALL ingredient labels EVERY TIME YOU BUY

Dijon vinaigrette

Makes 100 ml

3 tblsp red wine vinegar
2 tblsp water
1 tblsp olive oil
1 tsp Dijon mustard
¼ tsp garlic powder

Combine all in a screw top jar. Shake well to mix. Chill overnight to blend flavors.

Note: Will separate. This is normal. Shake before use.

Lime and coriander vinaigrette

Makes 200ml

2 tblsp red wine vinegar
2 tblsp lime juice
¼ tsp black pepper
2-4 tblsp coriander leaves, whole
1 clove garlic
1 egg yolk
1 tsp prepared mustard
150ml (¼ UK pint, $\frac{5}{8}$ US cups) salad oil
a pinch of salt
1 tsp lime zest (optional)

Put half the coriander and all the remaining ingredients except the oil in a blender. Process until smooth.

With the blender running, slowly pour in the oil until it's well blended.

Chop the remaining coriander very fine and stir into the dressing.

Coriander has a very strong taste; start with 2 tblsp and only increase the quantity if you want a stronger-tasting result.

This vinaigrette is an excellent marinade for ribs or fish. If you like a stronger lime flavor add 1 tsp lime zest to the blender as well.

CHECK ALL ingredient labels EVERY TIME YOU BUY

Mild blue cheese dressing
1-2 Servings

1 tblsp sour cream
2 tsp mayonnaise
2 tsp double (heavy) cream
1 tblsp blue cheese
1 tsp salad herb and spice mix

Mix all together and chill before serving.

Mock honey mustard dressing
1 Serving

1 tblsp Dijon mustard
1 tblsp mild coarse grain mustard
2 tblsp double (heavy) cream
1 tsp sugar

Mix all ingredients and serve.

Oriental salad dressing
1 Serving

1 tblsp sesame oil
2 tblsp canola oil
1 tsp sesame seeds
¼ tsp sugar
1 tblsp cider vinegar
Salt and pepper to taste

Mix all ingredients together.

Pepper and parmesan salad dressing
Makes 50 ml

2 tblsp sour cream
1 tblsp grated parmesan
2 tsp double (heavy) cream
1 tsp gluten free French dressing
fresh ground pepper to taste

Mix all together and chill before serving.

CHECK ALL ingredient labels EVERY TIME YOU BUY

Ranch dressing with blue cheese
Makes 375 ml

190ml (6 fl oz, ¾ US cup) sour cream
60ml (2 fl oz, ¼ US cup) mayonnaise
60ml (2 fl oz, ¼ US cup) double (heavy) cream
½ tsp salt
½ tsp black pepper
1 tsp garlic powder
1 tsp onion powder
1 tsp dried parsley
3 tblsp red wine vinegar
125g (4 oz) gorgonzola cheese, crumbled

Combine first 9 ingredients and 1 oz of the cheese and whisk well. Blend until smooth, then stir in the remaining cheese.

Spicy ranch dressing
10 Servings

275ml (½ UK pint, 1¼ US cups) mayonnaise
150ml (¼ UK pint, ⅝ US cup) double (heavy) cream
150ml (¼ UK pint, ⅝ US cup) cup water
1 tblsp vinegar
1 tblsp dried chives
2 tsp garlic powder
1 tblsp dried parsley
½ tsp paprika
1 dash cayenne pepper
1 tsp celery salt
½ tsp black pepper
1 tsp onion powder

Mix everything well and keep refrigerated.

Lemon dressing
Makes 650 ml

2 tsp salt
4 tsp sugar
450ml (¾ UK pint, 1 US pint) salad oil

CHECK ALL ingredient labels EVERY TIME YOU BUY

150ml (¼ UK pint, ⅝ US pint) vinegar
60ml (2 fl oz, ¼ US cup) lemon juice
1 tsp grated lemon zest
paprika
pepper

Combine all ingredients in a jar with a tight fitting lid and shake until well blended. Refrigerate.

Spicy blue cheese dressing
10 Servings

125g (¼ lb) blue cheese, such as Roquefort
150ml (¼ UK pint, ⅝ US cup) sour cream
150ml (¼ UK pint, ⅝ US cup) mayonnaise
¼ tsp pepper
a dash of gluten free hot pepper sauce
1 tblsp minced chives

In a small bowl, break up the cheese with a fork and mash it lightly, leaving some small chunks.

Add everything else but the chives and mix together thoroughly. Stir in the chives.

Cover the bowl tightly and store in the refrigerator for up to a week.

Classic vinaigrette
Makes 300ml

200ml (6 fl oz, ¾ US cup) olive oil
100ml (3 fl oz, ⅜ US cup) wine vinegar, cider vinegar or
    lemon juice
a little mustard powder or French mustard
salt and pepper
1 clove garlic, crushed
a pinch of caster sugar

Mix olive oil with wine vinegar, cider vinegar or lemon juice in a screw top jar. Season with mustard, salt, pepper, a crushed garlic clove and a pinch of sugar.

Shake well before use.

CHECK ALL ingredient labels EVERY TIME YOU BUY

Sesame (tahini) dressing
Makes 220 ml

60ml (2 fl oz, ¼ US cup) tahini
150ml (¼ UK pint, ⅝ US cups) water
2 tblsp lemon juice
half a clove garlic, crushed

Blend all ingredients until smooth. If you want it thicker you can reduce the amount of water.

Tahini yogurt dressing
Makes about 100ml

4 tblsp plain unsweetened gluten free yogurt
1 tblsp tahini
1 clove garlic, crushed
1 tblsp gluten free soy sauce
juice of ½-1 lemon

Mix all ingredients together and blend thoroughly. Store in the fridge, covered, for up to 4 days.

Bean salsa
4 Servings

400g (14oz) tinned black eyed beans, drained
3 tomatoes, chopped
1 tblsp chopped fresh coriander
1 small red chilli (jalapeno), de-seeded and finely
    chopped
2 garlic cloves, crushed
2 tblsp balsamic vinegar
juice and zest of ½ lime
salt and black pepper

Mix ingredients and refrigerate for half an hour before serving.

Rich vinaigrette
8 Servings

300ml (½ UK pint, 1¼ US cups) classic vinaigrette
60ml (2 fl oz, ¼ US cup) single cream

CHECK ALL ingredient labels EVERY TIME YOU BUY

Mix 5 parts classic vinaigrette with 1 part single cream by volume. Shake or beat well.

Blue cheese dip
4 Servings

125g (4 oz) blue cheese, crumbled
150ml (¼ UK pint, $\frac{5}{8}$ US cup) sour cream
150ml (¼ UK pint, $\frac{5}{8}$ US cup) mayonnaise
a pinch of garlic powder
a pinch of onion powder

Mix ingredients and refrigerate for half an hour before serving.

CHECK ALL ingredient labels EVERY TIME YOU BUY

RECIPES KIDS LOVE

Cheesy Thousand Island dressing
Makes 300 ml

250g (½ lb) cottage cheese
60ml (2 fl oz, ¼ US cup) gluten free tomato ketchup
1 tsp paprika
¼ tsp salt
1 tblsp relish
a pinch of pepper
½ stick celery
½ green pepper
2 spring (green) onions
2 tblsp olive oil

Dice celery, green pepper and onions finely.

In a blender combine cheese, ketchup, oil and spices.
Blend till smooth. Stir in remaining ingredients.

Chill for several hours.

French dressing
Makes 250 ml

150ml (¼ UK pint, $\frac{5}{8}$ US cup) salad oil
75ml (3 fl oz, $\frac{1}{3}$ US cup) red wine vinegar
1 tblsp lemon juice
1 tsp Worcestershire sauce
½ tsp salt
pinch sugar
½ tsp mustard powder
½ tsp black pepper
1 clove garlic, finely chopped

Mix together in a jar with a screw top lid.

Shake well before use.

CHECK ALL ingredient labels EVERY TIME YOU BUY

Ranch dressing

Makes 350 ml

190ml (6 fl oz, ¾ US cup) sour cream
60ml (2 fl oz, ¼ US cup) mayonnaise
60ml (2 fl oz, ¼ US cup) double (heavy) cream
½ tsp salt
½ tsp black pepper
1 tsp garlic powder
1 tsp onion powder
1 tsp dried parsley
2 tblsp red wine vinegar

Combine ingredients and whisk well.

Sweet vinaigrette

8 Servings

570ml (1 UK pint, 2½ US cups) classic vinaigrette
30ml (1 fl oz, $\frac{1}{8}$ US cup) mint sauce
30ml (1 fl oz, $\frac{1}{8}$ US cup) tomato purée
a pinch of paprika
60ml (2 fl oz, ¼ US cup) single cream (optional)

Mix the classic vinaigrette, mint sauce, tomato purée and
a pinch of paprika. If you prefer the richer tasting
version, add the cream. Shake or beat well.

CHECK ALL ingredient labels EVERY TIME YOU BUY

PRESERVES AND PICKLES

Fig preserve with brandy
Makes 4 standard jars

1 kg (2 lb) fresh figs
375g (12 oz) light brown sugar
1 tblsp lemon juice
3 tblsp brandy

Wash and prepare figs and cut into quarters. Put into a large heavy saucepan with the remaining ingredients. Stir well to mix.

Put pan onto a low heat and cook, stirring occasionally, for 1¾ hours until a thick, dark syrup forms and setting point is reached. To test for this, take a teaspoonful of the preserve and put onto a cold saucer. When it has cooled, push it with your finger; if wrinkles form when you prod it, the preserve is ready. Remove from heat, cool and pour into a screw top jar. When thoroughly cool, cover, seal and label.

Pears in orange syrup
Makes 4 standard jars

1.5 kg (3 lb) cooking pears
275ml (½ UK pint, 1¼ US cups) water
60ml (2 fl oz, ¼ US cup) orange Curaçao
1 level tsp cardamom seeds

Preheat oven to 180°C (350°F, gas mark 4).

Peel pears, cut in half and remove cores. Place side by side in a shallow baking dish. Combine water, orange liqueur and cardamom seeds. Pour over fruit. Cover dish with lid or foil. Bake for 50-60 minutes until tender.

Remove from oven and leave to cool. Carefully transfer pears into a large preserving jar and pour in cooking liquid, including cardamom seeds. If necessary top up with water or a little more orange liqueur. Label and store in a cool place.

CHECK ALL ingredient labels EVERY TIME YOU BUY

Winter chutney
Makes 1 kg

1 kg (2 lb) cooking apples, peeled and chopped
3 green peppers, de-seeded and chopped
60g (2 oz) raisins
juice of 1 lemon
½ tsp paprika

Mix ingredients together, blend until smooth. Store in an airtight jar.

CHECK ALL ingredient labels EVERY TIME YOU BUY

RECIPES KIDS LOVE

Cranberry relish
Makes about 1 kilo

275ml (½ UK pint, 1¼ US cups) dark rum or water
1 tsp grated lemon rind
185g (6 oz) sugar
250g (½ lb) walnuts, pecans or almonds – chopped
750g (1½ lb) cranberries

Heat sugar and rum in a saucepan to boiling point. Add cranberries and lemon zest.

Bring back to the boil and immediately lower heat so that the mixture is on a low, rolling boil, just above a simmer. Cover and cook for 10 minutes, stirring occasionally.

Stir in chopped nuts. Cook for a further 1-2 minutes, then remove from heat, cover and leave to cool completely.

The alcohol content all boils off during cooking, but if you would rather leave it out, just substitute an equal amount of water.

Lemon curd
Makes 1 kg

juice and finely grated rind of 4 lemons
125g (¼ lb) butter
500g (1 lb) sugar
4 eggs

Beat the eggs.

Place lemon juice and rind in a non-metallic bowl with the butter and sugar. Microwave for 1-1½ minutes until the mixture hot (not boiling) and the sugar has dissolved.

Add lemon and sugar mixture gradually to the eggs, beating thoroughly, then return mixture to the bowl.

CHECK ALL ingredient labels EVERY TIME YOU BUY

Put the bowl back into the microwave and heat in 30 second bursts, mixing thoroughly each time, until it becomes thick, glossy and smooth.

Leave to cool. Transfer to clean jam jars, cover and refrigerate for use within 3-4 weeks, or into plastic containers (leaving head space for expansion) to be frozen for use within 6 months.

Frozen lemon curd takes 3-4 hours to defrost at room temperature.

CHECK ALL ingredient labels EVERY TIME YOU BUY

DRINKS AND SMOOTHIES

Wassail
(Traditional Christmas carollers' drink)

4 bottles of wine
500g (1 lb) sugar
nutmeg
cloves
ginger
mace
allspice berries
cinnamon
12 eggs, separated
12 cooking apples

Bake the apples in a hot oven for about 45 minutes.

Mix the spices with the sugar and water. Bring to the boil, then pour in the wine to heat up.

Meanwhile, beat the whites until stiff. Beat the yolks separately and then fold into the whites. Pour on the spiced hot wine and mix well.

Add the whole apples.

Mango smoothie
8 Servings
900ml (1½ UK pints, 3¾ US cups) mango nectar, chilled
600ml (1 UK pint, 2½ US cups) plain gluten free yogurt
1½ tblsp honey
½ tsp mixed spice

Blend all ingredients together until smooth.

Chocolate soy milk smoothie
2 Servings
450ml (¾ UK pint, 1 US pint) soy milk
2 tblsp sugar
1 tblsp cocoa powder

CHECK ALL ingredient labels EVERY TIME YOU BUY

1 tsp potato flour
½ tsp vanilla essence

Dissolve the potato flour in a little water or soy milk.

Bring the soy milk to the boil.

Add the sugar, cocoa and potato flour mixture to the boiling soy milk. Boil on low heat, stirring continuously, for 2 minutes until smooth and thick.

Serve hot, or cool and refrigerate to serve cold.

Café frappé (Iced coffee)
1 Serving

About three quarters of a glass of milk
1½ tsp instant coffee dissolved in 1 tblsp boiling water
½-1 tsp sugar
1 scoop vanilla or coffee ice cream
Whipped cream (optional)

Combine all the ingredients except cream in your blender or smoothie maker and blend until frothy. Pour into the glass.

Top with whipped cream, if liked.

Mocha frappé

Add 1 tsp cocoa, mixed with the coffee and boiling water at the start of the recipe.

CHECK ALL ingredient labels EVERY TIME YOU BUY

RECIPES KIDS LOVE

Banana smoothie
Makes 4

570ml (1 UK pint, 2½ US cups) cold milk
1 very ripe banana, peeled and cut into pieces
3 tblsp gluten free vanilla or toffee ice cream

Place all into a blender or smoothie maker and blend until smooth.

Chocolate ice cream soda
1 Serving

2 tsp gluten free drinking chocolate
2 tblsp milk
2 tblsp gluten free vanilla ice cream
1 cup lemonade
1 ice cube

Blend drinking chocolate, milk and half the ice cream together. Stir into lemonade.

Pour into a glass, add the ice cube and the remaining ice cream. Serve with a straw.

CHECK ALL ingredient labels EVERY TIME YOU BUY

CELEBRATION AND PARTY SPECIALS: SAVORY

Chinese rice dumplings (T'ang-t'uan)
Makes 24

250g (½ lb) minced pork
2 tblsp gluten free soy sauce
½ tsp sugar
½ tsp sherry or Chinese rice wine
1 large spring (green) onion, chopped very fine
1 tblsp cornflour (cornstarch)
½ tblsp sesame oil
500g (1 lb) glutinous rice flour
150ml (¼ UK pint, ⅝ US cup) warm water

Mix pork, soy sauce, sugar, sherry, spring onion, cornflour and sesame oil together to make the stuffing.

Knead the flour into a dough with warm water and divide into 24 portions. Make them into hollow thimbles, put 1 heaped tsp of the stuffing into each, pinch together and roll to form a ball.

Bring 1.5 litres (3 pints) of water to boil in a large pot. Drop the dumplings in and boil for 5 minutes, timing from when the water starts to boil again.

When the dumplings float to the surface, add 300ml (½ pint) of cold water and boil for a further 3 minutes.

Serve a minimum of four to a bowl of clear soup. The juice inside will be very hot, take care not to scald yourself when eating them.

CHECK ALL ingredient labels EVERY TIME YOU BUY

Anniversary casserole

6 Servings

6 chicken portions
salt and pepper
2 tblsp oil
150ml (¼ UK pint, ⅝ US cup) orange juice
75ml (3 fl oz, ⅓ US cup) wine vinegar
275ml (½ UK pint, 1¼ US cups) cider or water
2 large onions, chopped
½ level tsp ground coriander
1 orange
1 banana

Skin chicken portions, season and fry on both sides until browned.

Place them in a casserole dish, add the orange juice, vinegar and cider or water. Add onions, season and sprinkle with coriander.

Cover and bake for about 2 hours until tender.

Peel and chop banana and orange and add to casserole. Bake for a further 30 minutes and serve.

Canapés

Makes about 20

4 sticks of celery
250g (½ lb) cream cheese with chives
2 tsp anchovy essence
pepper
a few olives (preferably stuffed)

Cut celery into 5cm (2") lengths and put into a bowl of iced water.

Slice olives for garnish.

Mix together cream cheese, anchovy essence and pepper.

Remove celery from the water, drain well and pat dry with kitchen towel.

CHECK ALL ingredient labels EVERY TIME YOU BUY

Fill celery pieces with cream cheese mixture and top each with a slice of olive.

Roast partridge

1 Serving

A young partridge, about 700g (1½ lb)
Strips of fat pork to cover
A knob of butter
salt and pepper

Roast young birds only, older birds are more suitable for casseroles. A young bird should have smooth, pliable legs and a plump breast.

Partridge should be hung for 7-10 days before plucking and drawing, to tenderize and flavor the flesh. When the breast feathers can be plucked out easily, the bird is mature enough to eat. Alternatively, you may be able to buy an oven-ready bird.

The usual size for a young bird is about 700g (1½ lb), which will serve one person. For this reason, partridges are usually cooked in pairs called a 'brace'.

Preheat the oven to 200°C (400°F, gas mark 6).

Cover the bird with strips of pork fat, season and put a knob of butter inside the body cavity.

Roast for 15-30 minutes, basting frequently.

Remove pork fat and cook for a further 15 minutes.

Traditional accompaniments are watercress, game chips and bread sauce†.

† not suitable for gluten free diets

CHECK ALL ingredient labels EVERY TIME YOU BUY

Roast quail

1 Serving

A young quail* about 250-500g (½-1 lb)
Strips of pork fat to cover
A knob of butter

Preheat oven to 210°C (425°F, gas mark 7).

Season bird, cover with strips of pork fat, put a knob of butter inside. Roast for 10 minutes. Remove pork fat and put back for a further 10 minutes.

Traditional accompaniments are watercress, game chips, fried breadcrumbs† and bread sauce†.

† Not suitable for gluten free diets.
* The young bird has pointed feathers, soft feet and short rounded spurs. It doesn't need hanging and is not drawn. It is served whole.

Roast grouse

1 Serving

A 1-1.5 kg (2-3lb) grouse
Strips of fat pork to cover
salt and pepper

Buy oven ready, so that the hanging, plucking and drawing will have been done for you. Only young birds are suitable for roasting; older ones make good casseroles, though. You can tell a young bird by its soft, even feathers, smooth pliable legs and plump breast.

If you have to do the game preparation yourself, the bird needs to be hung for 7-10 days, before it is plucked and drawn. When the breast feathers can be plucked out easily the bird is ready to cook.

Preheat oven to 200°C (400°F, gas mark 6).

Season with salt and black pepper. Cover with strips of pork fat and put a knob of butter inside. Roast for 30 minutes, remove pork fat, and roast for a further 15 minutes.

Traditional accompanimentsare Watercress, game chips, fried breadcrumbs† and bread sauce†

† Not suitable for gluten free diets.

CHECK ALL ingredient labels EVERY TIME YOU BUY

Roast pigeon

2 Servings

A young pigeon, about 700-1150g (1½-2½ lb) in weight
A knob of butter
Bacon to cover

Choose a young bird with rosy flesh.

Preheat oven to 190°C (375°F, gas mark 5).

Put a knob of butter inside and bacon rashers on the breast. Place on a rack in a roasting tin and roast for 15 minutes.

Remove from the oven, take the bacon rashers off and return the bird to the oven. Roast for a further 10-20 minutes.

Traditional accompaniments are Brussels sprouts, braised celery and bread sauce†.

† not suitable for gluten free diets

Roast goose

8-12 Servings

A 3-6 kg (6-12lb) goose

Preheat oven to 200°C (400°F, gas mark 6).

Prick bird all over. Stuff and weigh to calculate cooking time. Place on a rack in a roasting tin. Season with salt and pepper.

If using stuffing, include the weight of the stuffing when calculating cooking time. Roast for 35 minutes per kilo (15 minutes per lb) plus 15 minutes, adding potatoes around the bird about 1¼ hours before the end of cooking. There is no need to add any oil, as the goose will provide more than enough grease.

Half an hour before the end of cooking, remove foil and return to the oven to brown.

A good stuffing is Apricot and Rice Stuffing, based on rice, not breadcrumbs, or serve extra vegetables.

Traditional accompaniments are boiled onions and apple sauce.

CHECK ALL ingredient labels EVERY TIME YOU BUY

Roast pheasant

3-4 Servings

A 1.5-1.7kg (3½-4 lb) Pheasant
Butter to rub into skin
Bacon rashers to cover

It is best to buy an oven ready bird, so that the hanging, plucking and drawing will have been done for you.

If you have to do the game preparation yourself, the pheasant needs to be hung for 7-10 days, before it is plucked and drawn. When the breast feathers can be plucked out easily the bird is ready to cook.

Preheat oven to 200°C (400°F, gas mark 6).

Rub butter into skin and cover with bacon rashers. Place on a rack in a roasting tin.

Roast for 20 minutes per lb.

Traditional accompaniments: game chips and bread sauce†.

† not suitable for gluten free diets

CHECK ALL ingredient labels EVERY TIME YOU BUY

RECIPES KIDS LOVE

Roast saddle of lamb
8 Servings

5 kg (10 lb) saddle of lamb
1 large sprig of fresh rosemary
30g (1 oz) butter, cut into small pieces

Preheat oven to 180°C (350°F, gas mark 4).

Place rosemary on saddle, dot with butter and wrap in foil.

Place in a roasting tin and roast for 2 hours.

Fold back foil. Pour 1 pint of boiling water around the meat. Turn oven up to 200°C (400°F, gas mark 6) and cook for a further 40 minutes.

Roast duck
4-6 Servings

A 2-3 kg (4-6lb) duck

Preheat oven to 200°C (400°F, gas mark 6).

Remove the tail and discard. Prick the bird all over. Stuff and weigh to calculate cooking time. Sprinkle with salt and cover with foil. Put the bird on a rack in a roasting tin.

If using stuffing, include the weight of the stuffing when calculating cooking time. Roast for 45 minutes per kilo (20 minutes per lb), adding potatoes around the bird about 1¼ hours before the end of cooking. There is no need to add any oil, as the duck will provide sufficient grease.

Half an hour before the end of cooking, remove foil and return to the oven to brown.

A good stuffing is Apricot and Rice Stuffing.

Traditionally accompanied by a sweet sauce, such as apple, cranberry or Bigarade sauce.

CHECK ALL ingredient labels EVERY TIME YOU BUY

Roast capon

6-8 Servings

A 3-4 kg (6-8 lb) capon

Preheat oven to 150°C (300°F, gas mark 2).

Remove the little pads of fat just inside the cavity and put to one side. Stuff. Place on a rack, in a roasting tin, tie feet together and cover with the fat removed earlier. Sprinkle the legs of the bird with salt. Lay bacon rashers over the breast and cover the bird with foil.

Roast for 2 hours.

Remove from oven, surround with potatoes and drizzle them with oil. Return to the oven and roast for a further hour.

Remove from the oven, take the bacon and foil off (keep the bacon to serve with the meat). Return to the oven and roast for a final 30 minutes.

Use a stuffing based on rice instead of breadcrumbs, or serve extra vegetables.

Traditional accompaniments are bacon rolls, chipolatas, gravy and bread sauce†.

† Not suitable for gluten free diets).

Roast turkey

4-20 Servings

Allow 300-350g (10-12 oz) per serving

Preheat oven to 180°C (350°F, gas mark 4).

To prevent the breast meat from drying out, you can either buy a 'ready basted'‡ bird or insert butter‡ or finely minced pork between the breast skin and the meat. This requires some care, to avoid piercing the skin. If you want to do this, you need to ensure the breast stays covered during thawing, so that the skin does not dry out and lose its flexibility.

You need clean hands with short fingernails to succeed in releasing the skin from the breast meat. The method is

CHECK ALL ingredient labels EVERY TIME YOU BUY

to lift the skin and gently push your fingers between the skin and the meat, gradually releasing the skin from the meat until there is a pocket into which you can insert the butter or pork mince. Be careful not to tear the skin. If you take it slowly and carefully, you will find it is quite easy to do.

Once the skin is free, put a thin layer of butter or pork mince in, to completely cover the surface of the meat. Then pull the skin back down, and smooth it into shape. Sprinkle the bird with salt.

Alternatively, you can just cover the breast with strips of fat bacon, in which case you only need to season the legs and wings.

Weigh the stuffing mixtures and add them to the weight of the bird to calculate the cooking time. Stuff the neck and body cavities with the stuffings you have chosen. Add the bacon strips, if used. Wrap the turkey in foil.

Roast for 45 minutes per kilo (20 minutes per pound).

An hour before the end of cooking time, unwrap the foil to let the turkey brown and remove the bacon, if used. Leave pieces of foil over the ends of the legs and wings so that they do not scorch.

Traditional stuffings in the UK are sausagemeat and turkey liver stuffing in the body cavity (try sausagemeat and chestnut or parsnip stuffing for a lighter flavor), parsley and thyme† at the neck end. You can substitute finely minced pork for the sausagemeat, but the other stuffing will need to be based on rice or some other gluten free carbohydrate.

Traditional accompaniments are bread sauce†, chipolatas†, Brussels sprouts, roast parsnips and cranberry sauce (in US).

† Not suitable for gluten free diets.

CHECK ALL ingredient labels EVERY TIME YOU BUY

162 of 192 -

Roast sirloin of beef

12 Servings

3.5 kg (7 lb) sirloin of beef, boned and rolled
30g (1 oz) butter
1 tsp coarse sea salt

Preheat oven to 230°C (450°F, gas mark 8).

Rub joint all over with the butter and sprinkle with salt.

Roast for 30 minutes at 230°C (450°F, gas mark 8), reduce heat to 220°C (425°F, gas mark 7) and roast for a further 1¼ hours, basting occasionally.

CHECK ALL ingredient labels EVERY TIME YOU BUY

CELEBRATION AND PARTY SPECIALS: ACCOMPANIMENTS

Apricot and rice stuffing

Makes enough for a 2-3kg bird

100g (4 oz) cooked long grain rice
25g (1 oz) currants
25g (1 oz) nib almonds
25g (1 oz) onion, finely chopped
1 level tblsp chopped parsley
duck or goose liver, chopped (optional)
100g (4 oz) canned apricot halves
25g (1 oz) butter

This stuffing goes well with roast duck or roast goose, or indeed any fatty meat. Obviously, if using the stuffing with, for example, pork, you should omit the liver.

Mix rice, currants, almonds, onion, parsley and liver. Chop the apricots (the remainder of the can contents and the juice can be reserved to put into the gravy, if liked), and add with the butter. Mix well.

CHECK ALL ingredient labels EVERY TIME YOU BUY

RECIPES KIDS LOVE

Game chips
(Home made crisps/potato chips)
1-6 Servings

500g (1 lb) potatoes, peeled
deep fat to fry

Using a mandolin or other fine slicer, cut potatoes into very thin slices.

Pat dry on kitchen towel.

Heat oil, test by dropping a cube of fresh bread into the oil. If it browns quickly, the oil is ready to use.

Fry the chips a few at a time, so that they do not stick together.

Sprinkle with salt and drain well on kitchen towel.

Serve hot.

CHECK ALL ingredient labels EVERY TIME YOU BUY

CELEBRATION AND PARTY SPECIALS:
SWEET

Griestorte with raspberries
6 Servings

3 eggs, separated
125g (¼ lb) caster sugar
½ lemon, rind and juice
60g (2 oz) ground rice
1 level tblsp ground almonds
275ml (½ UK pint, 1¼ US cups) double (heavy) cream
1 level tblsp caster sugar
250g (½ lb) raspberries
icing sugar
angelica

Preheat oven to 180°C (350°F, gas mark 4).

Whisk egg yolks and sugar together until thick. Add lemon juice and rind, continue whisking until smooth and creamy.

Fold in ground rice, almonds and stiffly whipped egg whites.

Grease 2 x 20cm sandwich tins, dust with caster sugar and ground rice.

Divide mixture between tins, spread level and bake for 20-25 minutes. Cool and remove from tins.

Lightly whip half the cream, add caster sugar, fold in raspberries. Spread on one of the sponges and sandwich together. Dust top with icing sugar.

Stiffly whip the rest of the cream, pipe rosettes around the top and decorate with angelica.

Serve chilled.

CHECK ALL ingredient labels EVERY TIME YOU BUY

Caribbean bananas flambés

4 Servings

4 bananas
90g (3 oz) soft brown sugar
2 tblsp lemon juice
30g (1 oz) butter
2 tblsp dark rum

Preheat oven to 180°C (350°F, gas mark 4).

Peel bananas and cut in half lengthwise. Put into an ovenproof dish and sprinkle with the sugar and lemon juice.

Dot with butter and bake for 15 minutes. Transfer to a warmed serving dish.

Warm rum in a ladle, set alight and pour over bananas. Serve flaming, with cream.

Coeur à la crème

4 Servings

250g (8 oz) unsalted cream cheese
275ml (½ UK pint, 1¼ US cups) double (heavy) cream
1 level tblsp caster sugar
2 egg whites
250g (8 oz) raspberries or strawberries

Rub cheese through a sieve with the back of a wooden spoon. Mix with cream. Stir in sugar.

Stiffly whisk egg whites. Fold in to cream and cheese mixture.

Spoon into a non-stick heart-shaped mould, levelling top. Leave in the refrigerator overnight.

In the morning, turn out and decorate with raspberries or strawberries.

Serve with cream.

CHECK ALL ingredient labels EVERY TIME YOU BUY

Pavlova
6-8 Servings

Meringue:
4 egg whites
250g (½ lb) caster sugar
1 tblsp cornflour (cornstarch)
2 tsp lemon juice
¼ tsp vanilla essence

Filling:
250ml (8 fl oz, 1 cup) double (heavy) cream
2 bananas
1 small pineapple
2 passion fruit
2 peaches

Preheat oven to 150°C (300°F, gas mark 2).

Whisk egg whites until peaking. Add sugar a tablespoonful at a time, whisking until the meringue is very stiff. Whisk in the cornflour, lemon juice and vanilla essence.

Pile meringue mixture onto a baking sheet lined with paper and spread into a 23cm round. Hollow out the centre slightly and bake for 1½ hours.

Cool meringue, remove paper and place on a serving dish.

Cut pineapple in half and scoop out flesh. Remove the central core and discard. Dice the rest of the pineapple. Peel the passion fruit and peaches and slice. Peel the bananas and slice.

Whip cream until stiff and fold in some of the fruit. Pile into the centre of the pavlova and decorate with remaining fruit.

CHECK ALL ingredient labels EVERY TIME YOU BUY

Pineapple Romanov

4-6 Servings

1 large pineapple, with leaves intact
60g (2 oz) icing sugar
grated rind of half an orange
3 tblsp Curaçao or Cointreau
250g (½ lb) strawberries
275ml (½ UK pint, 1¼ US cups) double (heavy) cream

Cut pineapple in half lengthwise and scoop out the flesh. Cut out the central core and discard. Cut the rest of the pineapple into cubes. Keep the shells to one side.

Sift icing sugar and place in a bowl with the cubed pineapple and orange rind. Pour over the liqueur and leave to stand for 2 hours.

Set aside a few strawberries for decoration and slice the rest.

Whip the cream, fold in the sliced strawberries and pineapple mixture. Spoon into reserved pineapple shells.

Decorate with the reserved strawberries and chill for 30 minutes before serving.

CHECK ALL ingredient labels EVERY TIME YOU BUY

Café crème gateau

8 Servings

125g (4 oz) ground almonds
250g (8 oz) caster sugar
2 level tblsp instant coffee
4 egg whites
275ml (½ UK pint, 1¼ US cups) double (heavy) cream,
    whipped
icing sugar

Preheat oven to 190°C (375°F, gas mark 5).

Dissolve coffee in the least amount of boiling water possible. Stir in almonds and sugar and mix well.

Whisk egg whites until stiff, fold in the almond mixture.

Divide between two 18cm (7") loose bottomed cake tins. Level off.

Bake for ¾-1 hour.

Cool.

Sandwich together with the cream, sprinkle with icing sugar and serve.

CHECK ALL ingredient labels EVERY TIME YOU BUY

RECIPES KIDS LOVE

Easter truffle eggs
Makes 20

180g (6oz) plain chocolate
1 egg yolk
30g (1oz) butter
1 tsp coffee essence
1 tblsp cocoa

Melt the chocolate in a bowl over a pan of hot water.

Add the egg yolk, butter and coffee essence and mix well.

Leave in a cool place for 30-40 minutes.

Mould into small egg shapes and roll in the cocoa to coat evenly.

Put each 'egg' into a sweet case.

Variations:

1. Use milk chocolate, or a mixture of milk and plain.

2. Stir in a tablespoonful of chocolate sprinkles.

3. Use half and half cocoa and icing sugar for the coating.

CHECK ALL ingredient labels EVERY TIME YOU BUY

Fruit jelly meringue

6 Servings

Meringue:
2 egg whites
125g (¼ lb) caster sugar

Fruit jelly:
125g (¼ lb) granulated sugar
500g (1 lb) fruit (eg. blackcurrants, apricots,
    gooseberries or raspberries)
150ml (¼ UK pint, $\frac{5}{8}$ US cup) water
20g (¾ oz) gelatine, soaked in 4 tblsp cold water
150ml (¼ UK pint, $\frac{5}{8}$ US cup) double (heavy) cream,
    whipped
1 tsp grated chocolate (optional)

Preheat oven to 150°C (300°F, gas mark 2).

Whisk egg whites until peaking, then whisk in 3 tblsp of the caster sugar. Carefully fold in remaining sugar.

Put the meringue mixture into a piping bag with a plain nozzle and pipe tiny mounds onto a baking sheet lined with paper.

Bake for 1½-2 hours until golden.

Put granulated sugar and water into a pan and heat until sugar is dissolved. Add fruit and cook gently for 15-20 minutes until soft. Allow to cool a little.

Transfer fruit to a blender and blend into a purée.

Put the soaked gelatine into a bowl over a pan of hot water and stir until dissolved. Add to the purée and mix well. Leave until beginning to set.

Pour fruit into a 18cm (7") soufflé dish and leave in the refrigerator to set.

Turn fruit jelly onto a plate, spread with cream and top with meringues. Sprinkle with grated chocolate, if used.

CHECK ALL ingredient labels EVERY TIME YOU BUY

Gateau au chocolat

8-10 servings

200g (7 oz) chocolate (around 85% cocoa)
200g (7 oz) unsalted butter
200g (7 oz) caster sugar
6 eggs, separated

Pre heat the oven to 190°C (375°F, gas mark 5).

Break chocolate into pieces and melt in a bowl over hot water with the butter. Mix together until smooth. Leave to cool slightly.

Whisk egg whites until they are really stiff. Gradually whisk in the sugar.

Fold the egg yolks into the egg whites with a metal spoon. Fold in the chocolate and butter.

Pour into a buttered solid 22cm (9") cake tin.

Bake for about an hour, until a knife comes out clean.

Leave to cool.

For a real luxury treat, add a thick layer of chocolate buttercream frosting.

CHECK ALL ingredient labels EVERY TIME YOU BUY

Recipe Index

CHECK ALL ingredient labels EVERY TIME YOU BUY

CHECK ALL ingredient labels EVERY TIME YOU BUY

CHECK ALL ingredient labels EVERY TIME YOU BUY

CHECK ALL ingredient labels EVERY TIME YOU BUY

Printed in the United States
125994LV00010B/129/A